ALFRED L. HURWITZ, M.D.

Assistant Clinical Professor of Medicine
Stanford University, Stanford, California;
Formerly Assistant Professor of Medicine
University of California, San Francisco

ANDRÉ DURANCEAU, M.D.

Assistant Professor of Surgery
Department de Chirurgie
Université de Montréal
Hôpital Hôtel-Dieu de Montréal

JEAN K. HADDAD, M.D.

Associate Clinical Professor of Medicine
University of California
San Francisco, California

DISORDERS OF ESOPHAGEAL MOTILITY

VOLUME

XVI

IN THE SERIES

MAJOR PROBLEMS IN INTERNAL MEDICINE

Lloyd H. Smith, Jr., M.D., *Editor*

Illustrated by André Beerens, B.Sc.A.A.M.
Hôpital Hôtel-Dieu de Montréal

W. B. SAUNDERS COMPANY • PHILADELPHIA • LONDON • TORONTO • 1979

W. B. Saunders Company: West Washington Square
Philadelphia, Pa. 19105

1 St. Anne's Road
Eastbourne, East Sussex BN21 3UN, England

1 Goldthorne Avenue
Toronto, Ontario M8Z 5T9, Canada

Disorders of Esophageal Motility   ISBN 0-7216-4876-2

Last digit is the print number: 9   8   7   6   5   4   3   2   1

EDITOR'S FOREWORD

The gullet is not an organ of glamour or versatility. Even the name "esophagus" reflects by etymology its function of carrying food —from the pharynx to the stomach. In brief it is simply a conduit which transfers but does not modify the diverse solids and liquids which traverse its span of 20 to 24 centimeters. The esophagus has been much maligned, however, in being considered only a membrane-lined tube for gravity flow. It must propel its contents, widely differing in composition and consistency, through the low pressure area of the thorax into the abdomen, where pressures may vary considerably. Furthermore, it must impede inappropriate reversal of this flow despite the variables of posture and pressure. Occasionally, of course, reversal is appropriate, when emesis is a protective activity to empty the stomach. In order to carry out these functions, the esophagus has a specialized musculature. The process of swallowing requires the complex coordination of striated and smooth muscle through voluntary and reflex actions to propel food in the proper direction and to protect the respiratory system. The pharynx is a common conduit for food and air, and hazards exist in that anatomical fact.

Where there is physiology, there is pathophysiology. This holds as true for a comparatively simple organ, such as the esophagus, as it does for the intricacies of the central nervous system. Disturbances of motility in the esophagus are common and may result in distressing dysfunction and symptomatology. These abnormalities may be functional disorders limited to the esophagus, or they may represent esophageal involvement by a more generalized disease, such as systemic sclerosis. From the work of many investigators, sophisticated methods have been developed to measure normal and abnormal motility of the esophagus and to sort out in a rational way the types of disorders which occur. This is of great importance, since therapy and prognosis can be shown to depend on this selective definition of abnormal function.

In this monograph Drs. Hurwitz, Duranceau, and Haddad have called upon their own experience, as well as summarized the work of others, to present the current state of knowledge concerning the disorders of esophageal motility. The result is an authoritative review, but one which is crisply focused on the problems faced in clinical medicine. As such it is a ready source of information for the general internist, as well as for the gastroenterologist in specialty practice.

LLOYD H. SMITH, JR.

ACKNOWLEDGMENTS

There are several people without whose help this work would not have been possible. The constructive criticism of R. W. Postlethwait, Jacques Bruneau, and Gilles Beauchamps is most appreciated. The patient assistance of Jacinthe Desjardins and Pierre Stasse, as well as the continuous support of the library, audio-visual, and photographic personnel at Hôtel-Dieu de Montréal Hospital is gratefully acknowledged. Finally, the dedicated secretarial assistance of Christine Holland, Carry Halvorsen, and Barbara Raposa in typing the manuscript has been invaluable.

The financial support of Dr. Pierre Bois and Dr. Jean-P. Fauteux, respectively Dean of the Medical School and Chairman of the Department of Surgery at the University of Montreal, and of the J. René Ouimet Foundation and the Alice and Germaine Gastien Foundation is gratefully acknowledged.

ALFRED L. HURWITZ, M.D.
ANDRÉ DURANCEAU, M.D.
JEAN K. HADDAD, M.D.

CONTENTS

CHAPTER 1

INTRODUCTION

Since the original publication of *An Atlas on Esophageal Motility* by Code and coworkers in 1958,[1] a large amount of material has been published about esophageal physiology and pathophysiology.

Of particular importance is the development of several new instruments and techniques that have improved the quality of the esophageal motility tracing.[2] In parallel with these developments, a more sophisticated understanding has evolved regarding the limitations of both the manometric technique and its interpretation.[3] These advances have led to new concepts in the pathogenesis of esophageal disease. For example, the lower esophageal sphincter dysfunction characteristic of achalasia was fully appreciated only after the development of water-perfused esophageal motility catheters.

In clinical practice an esophageal motility study should be considered in any patient whose esophageal complaints are not readily explained by a structural abnormality. The study may be diagnostic in achalasia, symptomatic idiopathic diffuse esophageal spasm, and esophageal scleroderma. It may be useful in the differential diagnosis of chest pain. The preoperative assessment of esophageal motility provides the surgeon with physiologic data that may influence the approach taken and quantify the results. Finally, manometric evaluation of the esophagus enhances one's understanding of esophageal function in certain diseases such as esophageal diverticula, gastroesophageal reflux, and oropharyngeal dysphagia.

This book has two purposes: first, to present normal and diseased esophageal function through the use of manometric tracings and second, to provide a rational approach to the patient with esophageal motor disease. The interpretation of motility tracings is emphasized, and how to perform an esophageal motility study is described in precise detail.

Motor diseases of the upper esophageal sphincter, the esophageal body, and the lower esophageal sphincter are covered sequentially in separate chapters. Both primary and systemic diseases known to influence esophageal function are discussed. An effort has been made to consider all factors that influence esophageal motility (e.g., the influence of gastric cancer and medications on the lower esophageal sphincter). A final chapter on the therapeutic and adverse effects of surgery on esophageal function discusses recent developments in this rapidly changing field.

The intent of the authors has been to provide a sufficient understanding of esophageal motility. Such understanding should lead to a more systematic approach to the patient with a swallowing disorder.

REFERENCES

1. Code C. F., Creamer B., Schlegel J. F., Olsen A. M., Donoghue F. E., Andersen H. A.: *An Atlas of Esophageal Motility in Health and Disease.* Charles C Thomas, Springfield, Ill., 1958.
2. Pope C. D., Christensen J., Harris L. D., Nelson T. S., Motlet N. K., Templeton F.: Diseases of the esophagus (work group I). *In* A survey of opportunities and needs in research on digestive diseases. Gastroenterology, 69:1058–1070, 1975.
3. Dodds W. J.: Instrumentation and methods for intraluminal esophageal manometry. Arch. Intern. Med., 136:515–523, 1976.

CHAPTER 2

EMBRYOLOGY, ANATOMY, HISTOLOGY, AND CONTROL MECHANISMS

EMBRYOLOGY[1-9]

The esophagus appears in tubular form with the formation of the foregut at approximately the twentieth day after fertilization. The early esophagus then occupies the major part of the foregut between the stomodeum and the gastric dilatation.

Initially, the esophagus and the trachea are a single tube (Fig. 2–1A). In its proximal portion, the lateral and anterior proliferation of the laryngo-tracheal fissure forms the early trachea and larynx. More distally, lateral ridges build a septum between the anterior and posterior walls of the primitive gut (Fig. 2–1B). During the septation process, cells at the union of the septa undergo necrosis and form coalescent vacuoles. A collapse of the basement membrane then occurs, allowing a passive filling by mesenchymal cells (Fig. 2–1C). The separation of the trachea and esophagus is complete by the thirty-sixth day (Fig. 2–1D). While this separation proceeds, a rapid elongation of the esophagus takes place, mainly through the ascent of the larynx.[1, 2]

At the proximal end of the foregut, the endoderm and ectoderm fragment progressively to open the digestive tube. The surrounding mesoderm differentiates to form the various layers of the pharynx and esophagus. Striated muscle progressively spreads as an envelope around the primitive pharynx. At the 12.5 mm stage, the inferior constrictor muscle can be recognized.[8] At six weeks of gestation, the circular layer of esophageal muscle can be identified, and nerve cells appear just peripheral to this layer. By the ninth week, the longitudin-

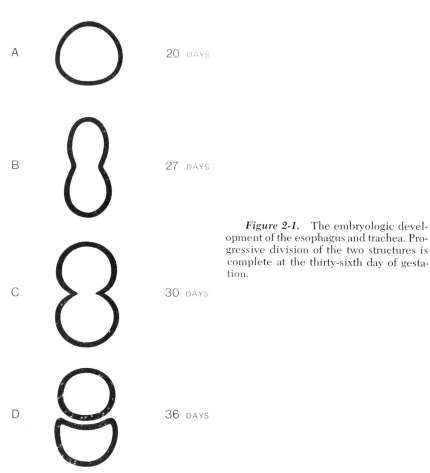

A   20 DAYS

B   27 DAYS

Figure 2-1. The embryologic development of the esophagus and trachea. Progressive division of the two structures is complete at the thirty-sixth day of gestation.

C   30 DAYS

D   36 DAYS

al muscle layer has covered the circular one. The muscular layer is a definite structure at 12 weeks.[3] Striation appears in the muscle of the proximal esophagus at a later stage than the somite period. This suggests that these striations originate from a primary differentiation of the esophageal muscle itself and not from pharyngeal extension.[4] The muscularis mucosae differentiates from a longitudinal myoblast layer at the same time that the longitudinal muscle layer appears.[5]

Blood vessels from the aorta and its branches penetrate the wall of the esophagus during the seventh week.

Innervation of the pharynx and pharyngoesophageal junction is based on the original branchial arches involved in their formation. The fourth arch is responsible for the formation of the pharyngeal constrictors and receives its innervation from the superior laryngeal nerve. The fifth and sixth arches give rise to pharyngeal and laryngeal musculature; they are innervated by the recurrent laryngeal nerve.[2, 9]

Neuroblasts from the neural crest migrate in the mesoderm adjacent to the endoderm of the foregut and form the myenteric plexus between the muscle layers of the esophagus. These cells are second-order or postganglionic parasympathetic neurons. Preganglionic neurons located in the mesencephalon and medulla oblongata originate from the neuroblasts of the neural tube. Through elongation the axons of these neurons will synapse with postganglionic parasympathetic neurons in the wall of the esophagus.[2, 9]

The gastroesophageal junction is the result of the coordinated development of the esophagus, stomach, and diaphragm and the innervation of these structures.

UPPER ESOPHAGEAL SPHINCTER (UES)

ANATOMY

At rest, the proximal esophagus is closed by a functional sphincter that creates a high pressure zone measurable by perfusion manometry[10] (Fig. 2–2). The cricopharyngeus muscle is classically described as responsible for this pressure zone. This muscle is attached anteriorly on both ends of the cricoid cartilage and encircles the proximal end of the esophagus as an uninterrupted muscular sling. Located at the level of the sixth cervical vertebra, the muscle appears as a posterior indentation on a barium swallow (Fig. 2–3). The extensive study by Zaino et al.[8] describes this muscle as independent of the esophageal musculature in most of the dissected specimens. In nearly one-third of the dissections, however, the muscle was fused with the longitudinal layer of the esophagus. Five specimens revealed no muscle distinction at the pharyngoesophageal junction. While the cricopharyngeus muscle can be identified as the extrinsic component of

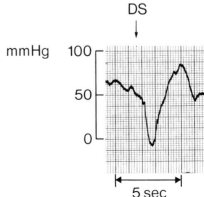

Figure 2-2. The proximal esophageal sphincter. A high pressure zone that is present at rest relaxes on swallowing. (*DS*, dry swallow.)

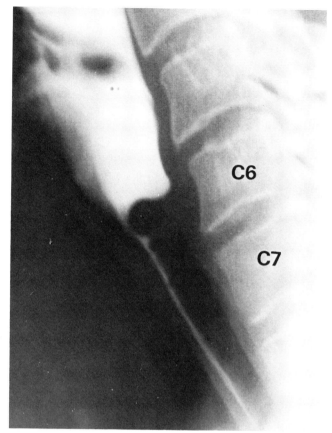

Figure 2-3. Posterior indentation of the cricopharyngeus muscle at the level of the sixth and seventh cervical vertebrae (*C*6 and *C*7).

the sphincter (Fig. 2–4A), the innermost circular muscle layer of the very proximal part of the esophagus may be the true intrinsic component of the UES (Fig. 2–4B). This circular musculature is attached to the suspensory ligament of the esophagus and was interpreted as a distinct muscular area in a large majority of Zaino's observations.

The main arterial supply to the proximal esophageal sphincter as well as to the cervical esophagus comes from the inferior thyroid arteries. Direct contributions from the aorta or from the carotid, superior thyroid, subclavian, and vertebral arteries are possible.[11] The veins from the submucous network drain through the wall of the organ to the peri-esophageal plexus and from there into the brachiocephalic vessels.

Lymphatic drainage from the proximal sphincter and cervical esophagus flows into the internal jugular system, the right and left lateral tracheal systems, and into the intertracheobronchial lymph nodes.[12]

HISTOLOGY

Histologically, the structure of the UES zone differs from that of the pharynx and cervical esophagus. Longitudinal sections of the pharyngoesophageal junction display a mucosa of squamous epithelium. In the submucosa, the muscularis mucosae appears immediately distal to the pharyngoesophageal junction and helps to delineate the cervical esophagus. A fibrous strand occasionally divides the cricopharyngeus muscle from the more distal circular fibers of the esophagus. While ganglion cells or intramural plexuses are not found in the cricopharyngeus muscle, a larger number are found in the transition zone of the circular musculature. These observations suggest the presence of a functioning sphincter in this area.[8]

INNERVATION AND CONTROL MECHANISM

Innervation of the upper esophageal sphincter is still poorly understood. The pharyngeal plexus, the superior laryngeal nerves and the recurrent laryngeal nerves, and all branches of the vagi probably provide the major motor innervation. Branches of the ninth nerve and the cranial branches of the eleventh nerve may also play a role (Fig. 2–5).

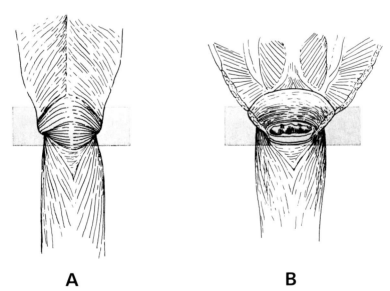

A   **B**

Figure 2-4. Anatomy of the pharyngoesophageal junction, posterior view. *A,* The shaded area includes the upper esophageal sphincter (*UES*) zone. *B,* After excision of the posterior hypopharynx and proximal esophageal wall. The shaded area now shows the inner circular muscle layer of the proximal esophagus. This layer may represent the intrinsic component of the UES.

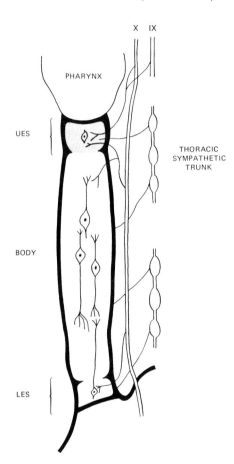

Figure 2-5. Innervation of the esophagus and its two sphincters, the upper esophageal sphincter (*UES*) and the lower esophageal sphincter (*LES*). Vagal fibers form the major neural supply (*X*, tenth cranial nerve (vagus nerve); *IX*, ninth cranial nerve.)

The upper esophageal sphincter is characterized by a high resting pressure zone that relaxes in a coordinated fashion to accommodate a bolus propulsed by pharyngeal contraction (Fig. 2–2). Closure of the sphincter creates a contraction, the initiation of the primary peristaltic wave. The resting tonic pressure zone maintained in the sphincter results from continuous stimulation by the vagus and glossopharyngeal nerves. During deglutition, inhibition of the discharges of these motor neurons causes relaxation. The interaction of these functions is coordinated through the medullary deglutition center. When swallowing occurs, a sequence of electrical stimuli to all the pharyngeal muscles creates an adequate propulsive pressure; simultaneous inhibition of tonic discharges to the sphincter causes it to relax. The motor nerves responsible for UES innervation are probably cholinergic, releasing acetylcholine at their nerve terminals.[13, 14]

BODY OF THE ESOPHAGUS

ANATOMY

The esophageal body is closed at both ends by the upper and lower sphincters. It is a muscular tube that measures 20 to 24 cm. from sphincter to sphincter. It may be longer in taller individuals. Lying anterior to the spine, it follows a slightly leftward course in its cervical portion and then curves back to the right in its middle third. From the seventh thoracic vertebra down to the stomach it again swings back to the left. The esophagus is under negative intrathoracic pressure throughout most of its course, except in the cervical and intra-abdominal portions. The aortic arch causes a small indentation at the junction of the proximal and middle third of the esophagus, and the distal third passes just behind the heart. The esophagus penetrates the diaphragm at the level of the tenth thoracic vertebra and reaches the stomach at the level of the eleventh. During its whole descent in the posterior mediastinum, the esophagus is surrounded by vital structures and can be influenced by their configuration and movement.

The arterial supply of the esophageal body comes from the terminal branches of the inferior thyroid artery in the cervical portion. Bronchial and paired aortic esophageal arteries penetrate the thoracic esophagus at the level of the seventh and ninth intercostal spaces. The intra-abdominal segment is supplied by the left gastric artery and by a branch of the left phrenic artery.[11]

The veins of the esophagus form an extensive submucous plexus that drains into the hemi-azygos and azygos systems. They permit venous flow between the portal and caval systems.

The lymphatics of the esophageal body drain to the intertracheo-bronchial or to the posterior mediastinal lymph nodes. Proximally and caudally the lymph flows toward the jugular nodes and the coeliac nodes respectively. The submucous plexus of lymphatics may drain submucosally for a considerable distance before perforating to the peri-esophageal nodes.[12]

HISTOLOGY

The wall of the esophagus is composed of mucosal, sub-mucosal, and muscular layers. There is no serosa. The mucosa contains a basal cell layer that sends dermal papillae toward the esophageal lumen. These papillae are covered by seven or eight layers of epithelial cells. The submucosa is a strong layer composed of connective tissue, elastic fibers, fibrovascular tissues, and a muscularis mucosae. The muscularis mucosae is a thin longitudinal muscular structure that begins just below the pharyngoesophageal junction and courses over the entire length of the organ. The muscular coat has an internal layer that is circular, while the external layer is longitudinal. The muscular coat is composed of striated muscle at the proximal end and of smooth muscle at the distal end.

Two types of nerve cells are present in the wall of the esophagus, the argyrophobe and the argyrophil cells. They are responsible for the intrinsic innervation of the esophagus and are located mainly between the circular and longitudinal layers of the muscularis. Afferent transmission of pain, pressure, and distention may be mediated through sensory endings in the submucosa.[15, 16]

INNERVATION AND CONTROL MECHANISM

The proximal striated muscle of the esophagus behaves like smooth muscle with a slow contraction and relaxation phase. The motor nerves to this striated segment are excitatory cholinergic and are integrated via the medullary swallowing center.[16, 17]

The esophageal body is composed mainly of smooth muscle. On stimulation, the circular muscle layer contracts at and above the site of stimulation while the distal muscle relaxes (the "on response"). On cessation of stimulation a peristaltic contraction starts in the previously relaxed esophagus (the "off response").[16, 17] The circular and longitudinal muscle layers appear to respond to cholinergic stimuli. A local control mechanism may be present to ensure coordination between the circular and the longitudinal muscle contraction.

The smooth muscle of the esophagus has a variety of excitatory and inhibitory receptors that have a physiological role in the modulation of the velocity and force of peristalsis.

LOWER ESOPHAGEAL SPHINCTER (LES)

ANATOMY

The gastroesophageal junction occurs at the transition line between the esophageal musoca and the gastric mucosa (Z line). In the majority of patients this squamocolumnar junction is observed 1 cm above the entrance of the tubular esophagus into the stomach.[18, 20] This junction is normally within the last few centimeters of the esophagus in its intra-abdominal position. The stomach forms a 70 to 80 degree angle with the esophagus at this point (Angle of His).

Longitudinal sectioning of the junction led a number of investigators to conclude that an anatomic sphincter was present at the esophagogastric junction.[20-22] Other studies, however, suggest that no such muscular thickening exists in the distal esophagus.[18, 19] Peters, in 2000

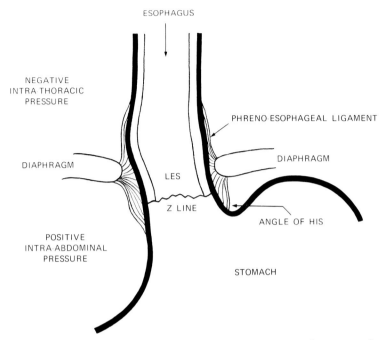

Figure 2-6. Gastroesophageal junction. The various structures known to influence the anatomic integrity of the area are shown.

specimens, did not demonstrate an anatomic sphincter at the esophagogastric junction.[23]

The esophagus passes from an intrathoracic position to an intra-abdominal one through the esophageal diaphragmatic hiatus at the level of the tenth thoracic vertebra. In this tunnel, the phrenoesophageal membrane originates circumferentially from the undersurface of the diaphragm, with contributing strands from the upper diaphragmatic surface. This membrane contains thick elastic fibers with little collagen and inserts into the esophageal musculature and into the submucosa from 2 to 5 cm above the squamocolumnar junction[24] (Fig. 2–6).

The arterial supply of the gastroesophageal junction comes from branches of the left gastric artery as well as from the inferior phrenic arteries. The venous drainage is via a rich submucous plexus connecting the portal system with the azygos system.[11] Lymphatics drain toward the posterior mediastinal, diaphragmatic, and coeliac nodes.[12]

HISTOLOGY

The mucosa at the gastroesophageal junction changes from squamous to columnar epithelium. It forms a mucosal plug or rosette that has been proposed as an antireflux mechanism. The submucosa contains muscularis mucosae that continues into the stomach. A sling of muscle fibers starting from the inner muscular layer descends on the lesser curvature of the stomach, forming a collar of muscle around the terminal esophagus. Bundles of smooth muscle cells form the muscular layer. Under electron microscopy, these cells have multiple areas of close and intermediate contact called nexuses. Nerve cells from the muscular plexus send their axons near the muscle cell surface, and the nexus allows transmission of electrical stimulation from one cell to another.[25]

INNERVATION AND CONTROL MECHANISM

The peri-esophageal vagal plexus around the distal esophagus converges into two trunks at the hiatus. Vagal supply to the distal esophagus and sphincter consists of cholinergic fibers and noncholinergic, nonadrenergic fibers. Innervation from the lower thoracic and coeliac sympathetic chain enters the esophagus in continuity with the vascular supply (Fig. 2–5).

The LES maintains distal esophageal closure and corresponds to an area of elevated manometric pressure. Experimentally, lower esophageal sphincter muscle responds differently to electrical stimulation than the muscular area immediately proximal or distal to it: relaxation occurs when the fibers are excited. LES muscle shows a steep length-tension curve that allows a more sensitive reaction to stretching. The resting tone of the LES is maintained through myogenic and neurogenic mechanisms. Relaxation is mediated by noncholinergic, nonadrenergic ("purinergic") motor fibers carried in the vagus. Contraction may be the result of adrenergic stimulation. Hormones may play a role in the neuromyogenic control of LES tone.[26–28]

REFERENCES

1. Smith E. I.: The early development of the trachea and esophagus in relation to atresia of the esophagus and tracheoesophageal fistula. Contr. Embryol., 36:43–49, 1957.
2. Gray S. W., Skandalakis J. E.: *Embryology for Surgeons.* W. B. Saunders Co., Philadelphia, 1972.
3. Jit I.: The development of the muscular coat in the human esophagus, stomach and small intestine. J. Anat. Soc. India, 5:1–13, 1956.
4. Jit I.: Development of striated muscle fibers in the human esophagus. Indian J. Med. Res., 62:838–844, 1974.
5. Jit I.: The development of muscularis mucosae in the human gastrointestinal tract. J. Anat. Soc. India, 6:83–98, 1957.
6. Barcsa A., Mohacsi L.: Development of the oesophagus under normal and experimental conditions. Acta Morph. Acad. Sci. Hung., 11:195–203, 1961.

7. Smith R. B., Taylor I. M.: Observations on the intrinsic innervation of the human foetal esophagus between the 10 mm and 140 mm crown-rump length stages. Acta. Anat., 81:127–138, 1972.
8. Zaino C., Jacobson H. G., Lepow H., Ozturk C. H.: *The Pharyngoesophageal Sphincter.* Charles C Thomas, Springfield, Ill., 1970.
9. Patten B. M.: *Human Embryology.* 3rd ed. McGraw-Hill Book Co., New York, 1968.
10. Winans C. S.: The pharyngoesophageal closure mechanism: a manometric study. Gastroenterology, 63:768–777, 1972.
11. Swigart L. L., Siekert R. G., Hambley W. C., Anson B. J.: The esophageal arteries: anatomic study of 150 specimens. Surg. Gynecol. Obstet., 90:234–243, 1950.
12. Rouviére H.: *Anatomie des Lymphatiques de L'homme.* Masson et Cie, Paris, 1932.
13. Doty R. W.: Neural organization of deglutition. *In: Handbook of Physiology,* (Code C. F., Heidel W., eds.) Sec. 6, Vol. 4. Williams & Wilkins, Baltimore, 1976.
14. Christensen J.: Pharmacology of the esophageal motor function. Ann. Rev. Pharmacol., 15:243–258, 1975.
15. Smith B.: The autonomic innervation of the esophagus. Clin. Gastroenterol., 5:1–13, 1976.
16. Christensen J.: The controls of esophageal movement. Clin. Gastroenterol., 5:15–27, 1976.
17. Diamant N. E., El-Sharkawy T.: Neural control of esophageal peristalsis. Gastroenterology, 72:546–556, 1977.
18. Mann C. V., Greenwood R. K., Ellis F. H.: The esophagogastric junction. Surg. Gynecol. Obstet., 118:853–862, 1964.
19. Bombeck C. T., Dillard D. H., Nyhus L. M.: Muscular anatomy of the gastroesophageal junction and role of the phrenoesophageal ligament. Ann. Surg., 164:643–654, 1966.
20. Byrnes C. K., Pisko-Dubienski Z. A.: An anatomical sphincter of the oesophagogastric junction. Bull. Soc. Int. Chir., 22:62–68, 1963.
21. Oglesby J. E.: The e.g. junction: two sphincters. Int. Surg., 60:135–139, 1975.
22. Lerche W.: *The Esophagus and Pharynx in Action.* Charles C Thomas, Springfield, Ill., 1950.
23. Peters P. M.: Closure mechanism at the cardia with special reference to diaphragmatic esophageal elastic ligament. Thorax, 10:27–36, 1955.
24. Strasberg S. M., Silver M. D.: The phrenoesophageal membrane. Surg. Forum, 19:294–296, 1968.
25. Daniel E. E., Bowes K. L., Duchon G.: The structural basis for control of gastrointestinal motility in man. 5th International Symposium on Gastrointestinal Motility, 141–151, 1976.
26. Rattan S., Goyal R.: Neural control of the lower esophageal sphincter. J. Clin. Invest., 54:899–906, 1974.
27. Christensen J.: The controls of gastrointestinal movement: some old and new views. N. Engl. J. Med., 285:85–98, 1971.
28. Goyal R. K.: The lower esophageal sphincter. Viewpoints Dig. Dis., 8(3), 1976.

CHAPTER 3

NORMAL ESOPHAGEAL MOTILITY

The esophagus is a muscular tube limited proximally by the upper esophageal sphincter (UES) and distally by the lower esophageal sphincter (LES). Its anatomy and innervation have been discussed in Chapter 2. Its function in propelling material from the mouth to the stomach is facilitated by complex, coordinated motor activity.

MECHANISM OF SWALLOWING

Normal swallowing involves both voluntary and involuntary motor activity. Swallowing is initiated by voluntary movement of the tongue. An involuntary peristaltic wave passes down the pharynx at a rate that is considerably faster than in the esophagus. When this peristaltic wave reaches the UES, there is a rapid, coordinated relaxation of that sphincter followed by a postdeglutitive contraction. An esophageal peristaltic wave that is propagated down the esophagus follows contraction of the UES. As this peristaltic wave approaches the LES, the sphincter relaxes. A postdeglutitive contraction in the LES occurs following the relaxation phase, with return to resting sphincter pressure after a variable period of time. With such normal peristaltic action being present, gravity is not necessary for the normal propulsion of the food bolus down the esophagus. Normal peristaltic activity is termed a "primary contraction" when a motor wave is initiated in the pharynx voluntarily, passes through the UES, and then moves down the esophageal body and through the LES in an orderly and continuous fashion.

PHARYNX

The recording of pharyngeal pressure and motility is usually not performed in routine manometric studies. This has been a difficult

14

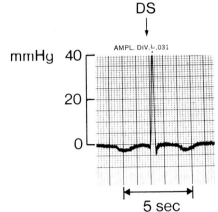

Figure 3-1. Normal pharyngeal contraction measured with a water-filled catheter. (*DS*, dry swallow.)

area to study with infusion systems because of the gagging that usually occurs with infusion of fluid into the pharynx and hypopharynx. The study of pharyngeal physiology is best done by using intraluminal strain gauges. Resting pressure in the pharynx is equal to zero atmospheric pressure. Utilizing intraluminal strain gauges, peristaltic contractions in the pharynx have been found to be as high as 400 mm Hg. The duration of contraction in the pharynx is brief, in the range of 0.2 to 0.5 second. The peristaltic wave travels rapidly through the pharynx (9 to 25 cm/sec).[1] Peristaltic pressure amplitudes recorded by infusion systems are usually much lower than those recorded by intraluminal strain gauges and are in the range of 20 to 80 mm Hg. (Fig. 3-1).

The pharyngeal motor wave is usually described as a single pressure spike, but an initial low amplitude pressure rise preceding the spike has been recorded, possibly caused by the propulsive force of the tongue. This early rise may actually represent the entering of the food bolus into the pharynx, since it seems more prominent when studied with a swallow of food.

UPPER ESOPHAGEAL SPHINCTER (UES)

The UES is a zone of high pressure with resting pressure greater than either pharyngeal or esophageal resting pressure. The sphincter is radially asymmetric in both its length and intraluminal pressure. Winans[2] has demonstrated that pressures (recorded by infused catheters) within the UES are greatest in an anteroposterior orientation (average 100 mm Hg) and least in a left-right orientation (average 30 mm Hg). These findings are consistent with extrinsic muscle (cricopharyngeus) contraction occurring mostly in an anteroposterior direction as opposed to intrinsic muscle contraction occurring uniformly

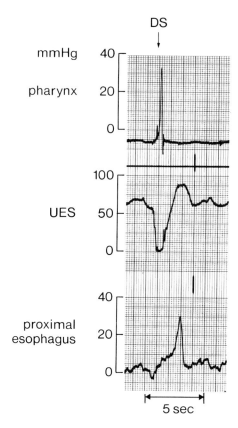

Figure 3-2. Normal UES function. Peak pharyngeal contraction occurs simultaneously with the nadir of UES relaxation. UES relaxation is complete to the level of the esophageal resting pressure. Contraction of the UES continues into the cervical esophagus as the primary wave of swallowing. (*DS*, dry swallow.)

throughout the muscle circumference. It appears that the pressures recorded in the UES are the result of both intrinsic and extrinsic muscle contraction. Elegant studies have recently been presented using computerized axial pressure recordings.[3] They graphically demonstrate the asymmetry of the UES. Because of this asymmetry, it is difficult to talk in terms of "normal" resting pressures. Unless precise tube orientation is known, comparative resting pressure measurements in the UES are meaningless. The problem of normal resting pressures in the sphincter might be better approached using an 8-lumen catheter assembly. Pope[4] has pointed out the difficulties of measuring sphincter pressure in an asymmetric sphincter. Averaging values of several pull-throughs may result in a mean pressure determination, which although convenient may be of no significance. Further discussion on this topic will be given in Chapter 7.

    Figure 3–2 demonstrates normal UES function. Resting pressure in the UES is greater than base line cervical esophageal pressure and demonstrates respiratory variation. UES sphincter length is variable but averages about 3 cm as recorded by infusion manometry. Coincident with pharyngeal contraction, UES relaxation to cervical esophageal base line pressure occurs in close to 100 percent of swallows in normal individuals.[5] Lack of complete relaxation to base line is abnormal and is seen in a variety of diseases (Chapter 7). Occasionally a transient low pressure rise is seen in the UES prior to the relaxation phase; it may represent the effect of tongue movement on UES pressure or drift of the catheter system into the contracting cervical esophagus with swallows. Not only must UES relaxation be complete, but it must also occur along with pharyngeal contraction in a coordinated fashion so that the swallowed bolus can enter the esophagus without resistance. Figure 3–2 demonstrates that the peak of pharyngeal contraction occurs simultaneously with the nadir of UES relaxation. Coordination occurs in virtually 100 percent of swallows in normal controls.[5] This relaxation phase in the UES occurs approximately 0.2 to 0.5 second after a swallow. Following UES relaxation a post-deglutitive contraction occurs in the sphincter with subsequent return to base line pressure. In the immediate infrasphincteric portion of the esophagus, a peristaltic contraction is seen to begin simultaneously with or briefly after UES relaxation (Fig. 3–2). This is the "primary wave" of swallowing.

Control of resting UES sphincter tone appears to be mediated via pharyngeal branches of the vagus and glossopharyngeal nerves. Relaxation is a result of inhibition of motor discharges, whereas contraction of the sphincter is the result of motor discharges of the vagus.[6]

ESOPHAGEAL BODY

Resting pressure in the esophagus reflects negative intrathoracic pressure, except in the most proximal 1 to 2 cm (infrasphincteric cervical portion) where pressures are closer to zero atmospheric pressure. Pressure in the esophagus varies with respiration, being lowest in inspiration (-5 to -10 mm Hg) and highest during expiration (0 to $+5$ mm Hg). The depth of respiration will be reflected in resting esophageal pressure oscillations, deeper breaths resulting in wider swings of pressure. Deeper inspiratory efforts will result in more negative pressure. Increased intrathoracic pressure, as occurs during the Valsalva maneuver, will be reflected in increased intraesophageal pressures (Fig. 3–3).

Esophageal peristalsis is a continuation of the pressure wave that has started in the pharynx and has traversed the UES. The esophageal contraction is usually preceded by a transient, minimal drop in pressure.[7] This may represent tongue or laryngeal movement or changes in respiration coincident with the initiation of the swallow. Peristaltic wave amplitude is greatest in the distal esophagus. A trough of diminished pressure amplitude has been demonstrated at the junction of the upper and middle thirds of the esophagus.[8] Peristaltic velocity is

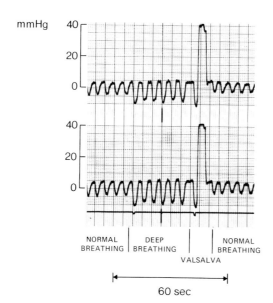

Figure 3-3. Breathing patterns in the esophageal body recorded at two levels. Deep breathing results in a decrease in intrathoracic pressure. A Valsalva maneuver results in a marked increase in intrathoracic pressure.

Figure 3-4. Normal peristalsis in the esophageal body. Following a wet swallow (WS), separation of the three wave peaks is shown by the three vertical lines.

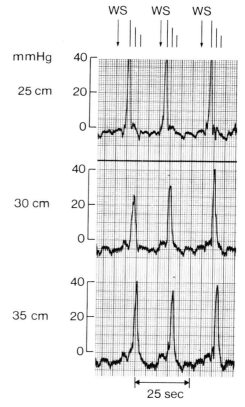

approximately 3 cm/sec in the upper esophagus, increasing to 5 cm/sec distally but slowing to 2 cm/sec just above the LES.[8] Figure 3–4 demonstrates normal peristaltic activity in the body of the esophagus. Nagler and Spiro, using uninfused catheters, performed serial manometric studies in young, healthy individuals and found variations in esophageal peristaltic pressures ranging from 20 to 90 mm Hg.[9] Although great variation was found between different individuals, serial studies in the same individual demonstrated reproducible peristaltic pressures. Primary peristalsis occurred in 90 percent of total swallows in this group. An increased frequency of nonperistaltic contractions was observed in these patients during periods of emotional upset.

Vantrappen,[7] also using uninfused catheters, found the amplitude of peristaltic peaks to be 28.6 mm Hg in the upper third and 37.5 mm Hg in the distal third of the esophagus, the durations of contraction being respectively 2.8 and 3.7 seconds. Pope,[10] using infusion rates of 2.4 cc/min, noted a higher amplitude of peristaltic contractions in normal individuals. Hollis and Castell[11] subsequently demonstrated that infusion rates as high as 15 ml/min may be required to give accurate estimates of peristaltic pressure and that then recorded amplitudes as high as 200 mm Hg in the distal esophagus are observed. Subsequent studies with intraesophageal transducers[8] have recorded amplitudes of 53 mm Hg to 69 mm Hg in the upper and lower esophagus respectively, with a pressure trough of 35 mm Hg at the junction of the upper and middle thirds. The amplitude and duration of the peristaltic pressure complex in young individuals has been shown to be significantly greater with wet swallows than with dry swallows.[12] Decreased amplitude of contraction but normal velocity in aged patients was shown by Hollis and Castell.[13] These data were in contrast to those found in elderly patients with diabetes and peripheral neuropathy, who in addition to this diminution in smooth muscle function also showed autonomic dysfunction in the form of increased tertiary contractions and absent peristalsis.[14] Table 3–1 summarizes the values for esophageal peristaltic pressures.

As stated above, normal peristaltic contractions initiated by a voluntary swallow are termed primary contractions. Secondary peristalsis refers to an orderly and propulsive wave that passes down the esophagus, not initiated by voluntary swallowing, but by local distention. Esophageal distention created artificially by an intraesophageal balloon or naturally by eructation may initiate a secondary wave. Tertiary contractions are usually spontaneous but may be initiated by voluntary swallows. These contractions are nonpropulsive in nature, may be single or repetitive, and may occur throughout the esophagus or in limited segments (Fig. 3–5). Although tertiary contractions are usually considered abnormal, they may occur in healthy individuals and may increase with advancing age,[14] although some dispute on this point exists.[13] Figure 3–6 demonstrates nonperistaltic contractions.

TABLE 3-1. *Pressure Amplitude of Esophageal Peristalsis*

REF. NO. (DATE)	NUMBER OF SUBJECTS	AGES OF SUBJECTS	LOWER ESOPHAGUS (MM HG)	MID-ESOPHAGUS (MM HG)	JUNCTION OF MIDDLE AND UPPER THIRDS OF ESOPHAGUS (MM HG)	UPPER ESOPHAGUS (MM HG)	TECHNIQUE
7 (1967)	25	47.5 (mean)	37.5 ± 1.24	35.5 ± 1.05	35.0 ± 6.4	28.6 ± 1.28	Uninfused Catheter
8 (1977)	10	22 (mean)	69.5 ± 12.1			53.4 ± 9.0	Transducer
9 (1961)	10	20–44		20–90 (maximal) 15–50 (mean)			Uninfused Catheter
10 (1970)	11		60–70		30–40°	50–70°	Infused Catheter
11 (1972)	10	25 (mean)	54–254 58–219				Maximally Infused Catheter
12 (1973)	10	21.6 (mean)	80–90° 60–70	65–75° 60–65	45° 42	60–65° 55–70	Infused Catheter {Wet Swallow / Dry Swallow}
13 (1974)	11 21	19–27 70–87	126 ± 14 77 ± 9				Transducer

*Values extrapolated from figures.

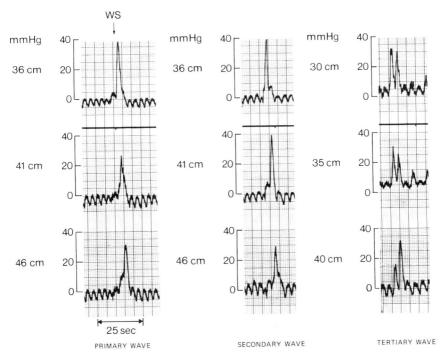

Figure 3-5. Primary, secondary, and tertiary contractions in the body of the esophagus. The primary wave is the normal response of the esophagus to voluntary swallowing. The secondary wave is a normal peristaltic wave that occurs in response to distension or irritation. A tertiary wave is not coordinated; it may appear spontaneously or after swallowing.

Note that such contractions may be simultaneous with others higher in the esophagus or may even precede them. In any event, the normal progression of the wave down the esophagus is not present. Figure 3–7 demonstrates nonpropulsive waves that are repetitive. Tertiary contractions, absence of motor response to swallows, and repetitive contractions may be the result of any number of conditions that affect autonomic pathways and that disrupt neural integration.

Control of esophageal peristalsis, described in Chapter 2, appears to involve a cholinergic excitatory mechanism.[15] With stimulation, the circular muscle layer contracts at and superior to the site of stimulation while the distal circular muscle relaxes (the "on response"). On cessation of stimulation, a peristaltic contraction starts in the previously relaxed esophagus (the "off response"). The smooth muscle of the esophagus has a variety of excitatory as well as inhibitory receptors that may have a physiologic role in the modulation of the velocity and force of the "off response" peristaltic complex.

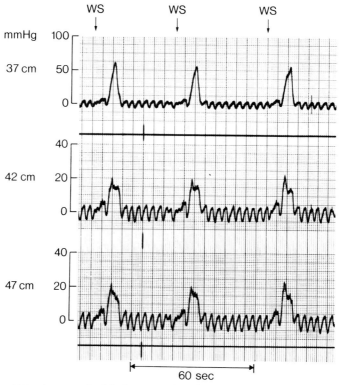

Figure 3-6. A nonperistaltic (nonpropulsive) contraction in the esophageal body follows voluntary swallowing (WS).

LOWER ESOPHAGEAL SPHINCTER (LES)

The lower esophageal sphincter is a zone of increased resting pressure, 2 to 4 cm long, which acts as a barrier to reflux of gastric and duodenal contents into the esophagus.[16] Conflicting views have been presented on this subject.[17] This high pressure zone has a resting pressure greater than either intraesophageal or intragastric pressure. Anatomic studies have failed to demonstrate any sphincteric muscle thickening at the esophagogastric junction in humans. The manometrically observed zone of increased pressure represents both intrinsic sphincter tone and extrinsic pressure from such surrounding structures as the phrenoesophageal ligament, sling fibers, and diaphragmatic crus.[18] The sphincter is radially asymmetric in both its length and pressure profile.[19] Thus, recordings from different arcs of the sphincteric circle will result in both different pressure profiles and different measurements of the length of the sphincter. Determination of "normal" values for sphincter pressure and length are therefore at best approximations and are usually the result of averaging the findings of several catheter "pull-throughs." The more determinations in different spatial orientations that are used to arrive at the mean value, the more accurate the result. It is difficult to compare sphincter pressure values unless the spatial orientation of the recording catheter is known. The greatest pressure recorded in the LES is in a left postero-lateral[18] or left lateral[19] direction, presumably because of the extrinsic musculature. The LES is in a resting state of tonic contraction and relaxes with electrical stimulation.

Resting lower esophageal sphincter pressure (LESP) varies from laboratory to laboratory and is dependent on technical factors. With infused catheters, the normal range of LES pressure is usually 15 to 25 mm Hg using the stationary pull-through method (SPT). Pressures recorded with the rapid pull-through technique (RPT) are 3 to 5 mm Hg higher.

Although some controversy exists as to whether or not LESP can be correlated with the presence or absence of reflux,[4] the majority of

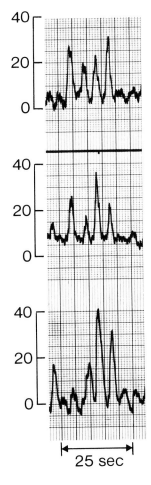

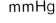

Figure 3-7. Spontaneous, repetitive nonperistaltic contractions in the esophageal body.

studies have supported the concept that a normal LESP protects against reflux.[16, 20] It is probably safe to say that patients with an LESP in the range of 0 to 5 mm Hg (incompetent sphincter) have a greater likelihood of refluxing at that time than do individuals with an LESP of greater than 15 mm Hg. Resting sphincter pressure is not constant and is under the influence of many variables (see Chapter 9). Likewise, reflux may occur intermittently in certain individuals, presumably at times when LESP is low. Figure 3–8 illustrates a normal LES with absence of reflux as demonstrated by an intraesophageal pH electrode.

During stationary pull-through studies, respiratory variation is seen in the LES. In the proximal portion of the LES, respiratory variation has the same pattern as is seen in the esophagus, negative with inspiration and positive with expiration. In the distal portion of the sphincter, however, respiratory changes are similar to those seen in the stomach, namely, increased pressure with inspiration and decreased pressure with expiration. The point where this shift in respiratory effect occurs has been called the point of "respiratory rever-

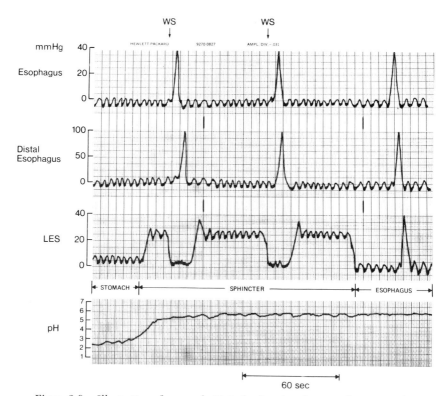

Figure 3-8. Illustration of a normal pH study, showing absence of gastroesophageal reflux as the normal LES is crossed. (WS, wet swallow.)

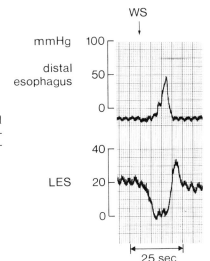

Figure 3-9. Normal lower esophageal sphincter (*LES*). Relaxation of sphincter anticipates the oncoming peristaltic wave. A contraction occurs after relaxation.

sal." Dodds[21] indicates that respiratory variation seen in the LES is probably the result of respiratory movement relative to the stationary catheter, rather than the result of an intracavitary pressure difference between the thoracic and abdominal cavities. He suggests eliminating the respiratory artifact by using the rapid pull-through technique (RPT).

Relaxation of the resting sphincter occurs as the peristaltic wave reaches the LES. LES relaxation occurs 1.5 to 2.5 seconds after the swallow is initiated. Figure 3–9 demonstrates normal LES relaxation. When the peristaltic wave crosses the sphincter, a postdeglutitive contraction occurs in the LES. This contraction follows the relaxation period. There is a return to resting sphincter tone following this contraction. Coordination between the oncoming esophageal peristaltic wave and LES relaxation is necessary for normal sphincter function. Likewise, relaxation in the LES must be complete, with pressure dropping to the gastric base line level. Abnormalities in LES relaxation and coordination will be discussed in subsequent chapters.

VARIABLES AFFECTING LOWER ESOPHAGEAL SPHINCTER PRESSURE (LESP)

When discussing normal values for LESP, one must take into consideration the many factors that affect this pressure. Pressure in the sphincter is not constant but probably varies considerably from moment to moment. Discussion of the factors that affect LESP will be found in Chapter 9.

REFERENCES

1. Dodds W. J., Hogan W. J., Lydon S. B., et al: Quantitation of pharyngeal motor function in normal human subjects. J. Appl. Physiol., 39:692–696, 1975.
2. Winans C. S.: The pharyngoesophageal closure mechanism: a manometric study. Gastroenterology, 63:768–777, 1972.
3. Welch R. W., Luckmann K.: The upper esophageal sphincter (UES) in man: significance of radial asymmetry and precise measurement of closure strength. Gastroenterology, 72:1168, 1977 (abst.)
4. Pope C. E. 2nd: Editorial: is LES enough? Gastroenterology, 71:328–329, 1976.
5. Hurwitz A. L., Nelson J. A., Haddad J. K.: Oropharyngeal dysphagia. Manometric and esophagraphic findings. Am. J. Dig. Dis., 31:313–324, 1975.
6. Christensen J.: Pharmacology of the esophageal motor function. Ann. Rev. Pharmacol., 15:243–258, 1975.
7. Vantrappen G., Hellemans J.: Studies on the normal deglutition complex. Am. J. Dig. Dis., 12:255–266, 1967.
8. Humphries T. J., Castell D. O.: Pressure profile of esophageal peristalsis in normal humans as measured by direct intraesophageal transducers. Am. J. Dig. Dis., 22:641–645, 1977.
9. Nagler R., and Spiro H. M.: Serial esophageal motility studies in asymptomatic young subjects. Gastroenterology, 41:371–379, 1961.
10. Pope C. E. 2nd: Effect of infusion on force of closure measurements in the esophagus. Gastroenterology, 58:616–624, 1970.
11. Hollis, J. B., Castell D. O.: Amplitude of esophageal peristalsis as determined by rapid infusion. Gastroenterology, 63:417–422, 1972.
12. Dodds W. J., Hogan W. J., Reed D. P., Stewart E. T., Arndorfer R. C.: A comparison between primary peristalsis following wet and dry swallows. J. Appl. Physiol., 35:851–857, 1973.
13. Hollis J. B., Castell D. O.: Esophageal function in elderly men. A new look at "presbyesophagus." Ann. Int. Med., 80:371–374, 1974.
14. Soergel K. H., Zboralski F. F., Amberg J. R.: Presbyesophagus. Esophageal manometry in nonagenarians. J. Clin. Invest., 43:1472–1479, 1964.
15. Diamant N. E., El-Sharkawy T.: Neural control of esophageal peristalsis. Gastroenterology, 72:546–556, 1977.
16. Fisher R. S., Malmud L. S., Roberts G. S., Lobis I. F.: The lower esophageal sphincter as a barrier to gastroesophageal reflux. Gastroenterology, 72:19–22, 1977.
17. Pope C. E. 2nd: Pathophysiology and diagnosis of reflux esophagitis. Gastroenterology, 70:445–454, 1976.
18. Winans C. S.: Manometric asymmetry of the lower esophageal high-pressure zone. Am. J. Dig., 22:348–354, 1977.
19. Luckmann K., Welch R. W.: The significance of lower esophageal sphincter asymmetry in man and its correlation with a new measure of closure strength. Gastroenterology, 72:1091, 1977 (abst.).
20. Haddad J. K.: Relation of gastroesophageal reflux to yield sphincter-pressures. Gastroenterology, 58:175–184, 1970.
21. Dodds W. J., Hogan W. J., Steff J. J., Miller W. N., Lydon S. B., Arndorfer R. C.: A rapid pull-through technique for measuring lower esophageal sphincter pressure. Gastroenterology, 68:437–443, 1975.

CHAPTER 4

ESOPHAGEAL MANOMETRIC TECHNIQUES

INTRODUCTION AND HISTORY

Measurement of intraluminal pressure, when performed simultaneously from different points in the esophagus, permits an evaluation of movement (i.e., motility). Manometry was first employed as a research tool in the study of esophageal physiology but has since become an important clinical tool for the understanding of pathologic states of the esophagus. Motor function of the esophagus was first studied by Kronecker and Meltzer in 1883.[1] They used small, partially inflated balloons to measure intraesophageal pressure phenomena. At that time the balloon size was considered important. Too large a balloon could stimulate motor waves in the esophagus. As early as 70 years ago, miniature electromagnetic pressure transducers were developed and used to measure intraluminal pressure directly. Because of its size, only one transducer could be swallowed at a time, and pressures at only one point could be obtained. Because of this limitation, open-tipped catheters were glued together to form a bundle of three or four that could be easily swallowed. Openings were made at different points in the catheters so that simultaneous pressure recordings from these areas gave an appreciation of "motility." These catheters were fluid-filled so pressures could be transmitted through the water column to the attached pressure-recording transducers. Catheters required intermittent "flushing" with water-filled syringes to ensure that recordings were not "damped." Recordings of intraesophageal pressure by fluid-filled open-tipped catheters gave recordings similar to those obtained by "distal" transducers, and the use of these catheters became popular in about 1950.

It became apparent by the late 1950's that there was variability in pressure recordings depending on what type of equipment was used (open-tipped catheter, fluid-filled balloon, or distal transducer) and that recorded pressures were not always an accurate reflection of intraesophageal pressure. Studies in 1952 by Quigley and Brody[2] and in 1959 by Pert et al.[3] convincingly demonstrated that constant perfusion of open-tipped catheters by external "bleeders" gave a more accurate measurement of intraluminal pressure. Resultant recordings more closely approached true intraluminal pressures and eliminated damping of tracings (caused by air bubbles in the system, plugs of mucus in catheters, or occlusion of the catheter opening by the luminal wall). Constantly perfused open-tipped catheters have been in common use during the last decade. More recently, tiny distal transducers small enough to allow a patient to swallow a catheter assembly containing three of these transducers have been developed. Their popularity appears to be increasing because of their ease of operation and apparent technical advantages.

GENERAL PRINCIPLES

Esophageal manometry attempts to measure intraluminal pressure events as accurately as possible by means of pressure-sensitive transducers. These transducers may be either distal (measuring pressure directly within the lumen) or proximal (measuring pressure transmitted through a water column from an opening in a catheter within the lumen). Transducer output is transmitted through preamplifiers to a recorder. Manometric data is then transferred to moving paper that gives a continuous record of pressure changes with time. When recordings are made simultaneously from different levels of the esophagus, one can gain an appreciation of movement in the organ. If both the distance between recording points is known as well as the recording paper speed, one can then determine the rate of esophageal movement.

PROXIMAL TRANSDUCER SYSTEMS

The proximal transducer system of pressure recording is the most commonly used at the present time. Intraesophageal pressure is exerted distally on an opening in a catheter and transmitted proximally through the column of water present in the catheter. Pressure is measured by a transducer located at the proximal end of the catheter and is electrically transmitted to the recording device.

TUBING

Current practice in many motility laboratories is to construct one's own catheters. The most common material used at present is thin-walled polyvinyl tubing. For consistency in results, tubing of the same diameter should be used for all studies performed in a given laboratory. At the present time, several firms are manufacturing stand-ardized catheter assemblies.

When catheters are constructed, the distal end is sealed, and a side opening is made just proximal to the sealed end. This will result in pressures exerted at the opening being transmitted up the tubing. A catheter assembly can be designed with as many tubes as desired and with openings at different points. The most commonly used grouping of catheters for clinical studies is one that contains three tubes with openings at 5 cm intervals, radially oriented 120 degrees apart (Fig. 4–1A). Any distance between openings can be selected, however, depending on the need. Note that when an opening is made in a catheter, the catheter is sealed off just distal to the opening. A solvent, such as tetrahydrofuran, is commonly used as a sealant on the ends of the catheters and as a glue to join the catheter assemblies. This

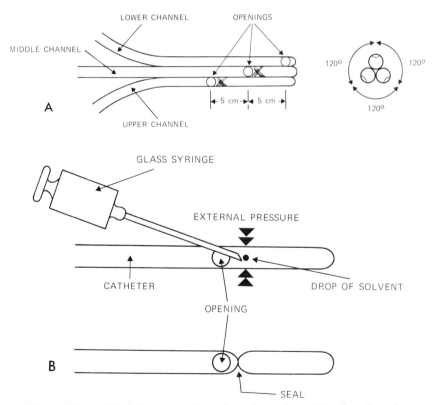

Figure 4-1. A, Triple lumen esophageal motility catheter. The three lateral open-ings are separated from each other by 5 cm and are axially oriented at 120 degrees. The crosshatchings represent sealing of the lumen distal to the openings. B, Manufacture of an esophageal motility tube. The lumen distal to the lateral orifice is sealed using a plastic solvent.

solvent acts rapidly. Minute amounts of the solvent are squeezed out from a glass syringe through a small-bore needle and through the previously made opening in the polyvinyl tubing. The lumen is simultaneously occluded using a small forceps applied externally to the tubing (Fig. 4–1B). Exerting forceps pressure for a few minutes is sufficient to allow the solvent to harden and to effect a permanent seal. Drops of tetrahydrofuran are also used to glue the tubing together along its course to make the catheter assembly. Nontoxic paint is used to mark the assembly at 1 cm intervals.

The proximal end of each catheter is fitted with a metal adapter so that it can be attached to a pressure-sensitive transducer by a three-way stopcock. This arrangement permits the attachment of an infusion pump through the side arm. One of the more commonly used transducers in present use is the Statham P23d, which has a response curve making it suitable to transmit the pressure ranges and rates of pressure change that occur in the esophagus (Fig. 4–2).

Transmission of pressure in such an open-tipped catheter arrangement requires that the tubing be fluid-filled so that intraluminal pressures exerted at the distal opening can be accurately transmitted to the transducer via the inelastic water column.

PERFUSION

A common artefact in manometric tracings has been that of damping caused by air bubbles in the system, by plugging of the catheters with mucus or debris, or by occlusion of the distal opening by esophageal mucosa. Damping was a constant problem in the 1950's and 1960's and was partially corrected by intermittent "flushing" of catheters. Recording inconsistencies were recognized when these intermittently flushed, fluid-filled catheters were used. After initial reports described constant perfusion of catheters,[2, 3] Winans and Harris[4] and Pope[5] demonstrated that constant perfusion gave more accurate estimates of intraluminal pressure and allowed for better differentiation

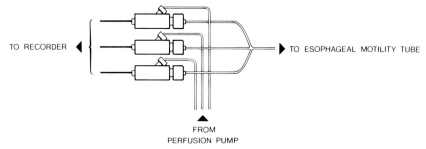

TO RECORDER

TO ESOPHAGEAL MOTILITY TUBE

FROM
PERFUSION PUMP

Figure 4-2.   Perfused catheter assembly. The fluid-filled tubing allows intraluminal pressure to be transmitted to the transducer membrane.

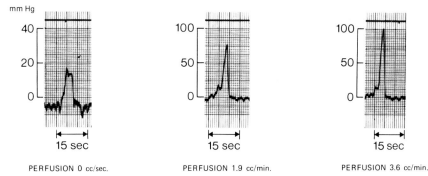

Figure 4-3. The effect of increasing the perfusion rate on measurement of the wave pressure in the esophageal body. As the perfusion is increased, wave amplitude increases. In addition, the change in pressure with respect to time ($\Delta P/\Delta T$) increases.

between the competent and incompetent lower esophageal sphincter.

Using a sphincter model, Pope[5] showed that fluid-filled balloons of varying sizes as well as uninfused open-tipped catheters consistently underestimated true pressures. In contrast, infused catheters more accurately reproduced true pressures in the model.

Studies were initially done with water infusion pumps giving flow rates in the range of 0.5 to 1.4 ml/min. Flow rates of this magnitude were shown not to affect base line pressures and to reproduce sphincter pressures accurately without damping. More recently, Pope[6] and Hollis[7] have shown that higher infusion rates are necessary to record accurately the amplitude of esophageal peristalsis. Higher flow rates are especially necessary when more forceful contractions occur, in order to prevent damping or pump artefact (Fig. 4–3). High infusion rates are also necessary to record rapidly changing pressures (high $\Delta P/\Delta T$).

DISTAL TRANSDUCER SYSTEMS

In the distal transducer pressure recording system, intraluminal pressure is measured directly by a distally located transducer. Electrical transmission to the recorder is via wiring in the solid catheter. Miniature transducers have been developed of such size that pressure can be recorded simultaneously from three sites. The advantage of these distal transducers is that perfusion is not necessary and that more accurate reproduction of intraluminal pressure is possible. The pressure response of these transducers virtually eliminates damping, even with such rapid changes in pressure as are seen with very forceful contractions (high $\Delta P/\Delta T$). The disadvantage of these catheters has been, to date, their relatively high purchase price and cost of repair. Durability was a problem with early models, and the sturdiness of the newer units remains to be determined. They are not yet in common use but may become popular in the future. A minor disadvantage is that they have fixed distances between transducers and are less versatile than catheters that can be made with openings at any interval desired.

RECORDERS

There are many polygraph recording devices in use at the present time. They vary usually from four to eight channels in recording ability. Most have some degree of versatility, allowing simultaneous recording of any number of pressure channels, respiratory or swallowing excursions, and intraluminal pH.

These recorders may be direct ink writing or heat stylus writing or may inscribe on photographic paper. Direct ink writers have the advantage that intraluminal events are inscribed on the moving paper immediately, whereas a brief time lag occurs before these events are seen on photographic recording paper. Some photographic recorders, however, incorporate an oscilloscope, and thus provide direct visualization of pressure. The delicacy of the mechanism that delivers ink to the pen nib necessitates meticulous care and cleaning of the direct ink writing systems. Ink and heat stylus recordings make good permanent records. Continuous exposure of the photographic recordings to light over extended time periods may result in "gray" paper with loss of recording contrast. Photographic recordings must be stored in the dark to prevent such loss of contrast. Ink and heat stylus recordings require no special storage precautions.

TABLE 4–1. *Variables Affecting Pressure Recordings*

A. VARIABLES ASSOCIATED WITH PERFUSED OPEN-TIPPED CATHETERS
1. Catheter diameter
2. Catheter length
3. Infusion rate
4. Mechanical factors
   a. Type of pump
   b. Inherent system drag
   c. Elasticity of tubing

B. OTHER VARIABLES
1. Spatial variables
2. Respiratory variation
3. Artefacts
4. Dry vs. wet swallows
5. Intraobserver and interobserver variables
6. Drugs, foods, hormones, and emotions

VARIABLES AFFECTING PRESSURE RECORDINGS

No standardization of manometric data presently exists. Variations in equipment and techniques from laboratory to laboratory have resulted in data that are difficult to compare. Any number of variables have been found that affect recording fidelity (Table 4–1).

VARIABLES ASSOCIATED WITH PERFUSED OPEN-TIPPED CATHETERS

1. Catheter Diameter. Kaye[8] and Lydon[9] showed that increasing the size of the catheter assembly diameter resulted in increased pressure recording in the lower esophagel sphincter. Individual catheter diameters were the same, but the diameter of the total catheter assembly was varied. They postulated that lower esophageal sphincter pressure (LESP) recorded with perfused catheters was, in effect, measurement of the resistance to stretch of sphincteric smooth muscle.

Another experiment varied individual internal catheter diameters.[10] The internal diameter of recording catheters was varied from 0.8 to 2.0 mm at varying infusion rates. Responses to different pressure amplitudes were recorded. As catheter internal diameter increased, recorded pressures increased for given infusion rates.

2. Catheter Length. Increasing the length of a catheter system increases the "drag" on the system and will decrease recorded pressures.

3. Infusion Rate. Infusion rates used in manometry studies vary considerably. Pope[6] found that low infusion rates (0.6 cc/min) used in earlier studies of LESP were inadequate to reproduce peaks of esophageal body pressure during high amplitude peristaltic waves. Although LESP may be accurately reproduced at these low infusion rates, peristaltic waves with amplitudes in the range of 100 to 200 mm Hg will be damped unless infusion rates are increased considerably. Rates as high as 10 cc/min may be required to record properly these forceful contractions.[7] Smaller diameter catheters require lower infusion speeds.

One of the most dramatic consequences of catheter perfusion rate has been in the study of the esophageal sphincters (Fig. 4–4A, 4–4B, 4–4C). The better understanding of the sphincter dysfunction occurring in achalasia was a direct consequence of catheter perfusion. Older studies had indicated that LESP was low in achalasia, without relaxation with swallows. This inaccurate impression was actually caused by damping of the catheter opening by a high pressure sphincter. Perfusion studies have demonstrated a high resting pressure with partial relaxation following a swallow. Figure 4–4C illustrates the effect of infusion rate on the LES in a patient with achalasia.

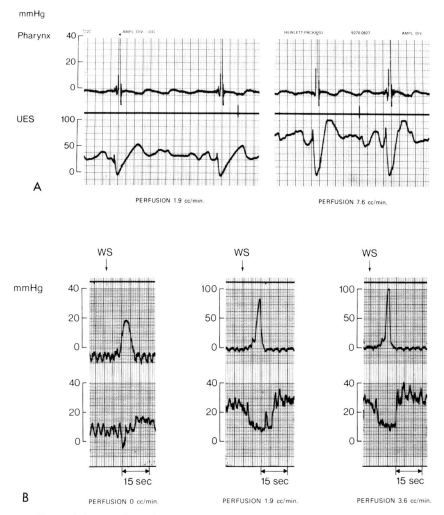

Figure 4-4. *A*, Effect of perfusion rate on the upper esophageal sphincter (*UES*) recording. At lower perfusion rates, the resting and postdeglutitive UES pressures are artefactually lower. In addition, the rate of UES contraction is slower. *B*, Effect of perfusion rate on the lower esophageal sphincter (*LES*). Without infusion, LES pressure is reduced, and the relaxation phase is difficult to assess. (*WS*, wet swallow.) *C*, Illustration of the effect of infusion rate on the LES in a patient with achalasia. When perfusion is stopped, damping occurs, and resting pressure drops without apparent relaxation following a swallow. (*WS*, wet swallow.)

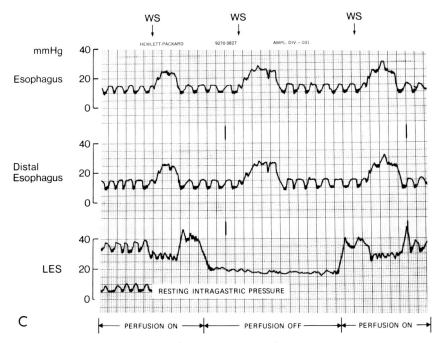

Figure 4-4 Continued.

Where the infusion pump is stopped, damping occurs and resting pressure drops without apparent relaxation following a swallow. Reinstitution of perfusion again demonstrates a high pressure, incompletely relaxing sphincter.

4. Mechanical Variables. The ideal infusion system should give a constant, pulseless flow of fluid delivered by a frictionless pump. Various pumps are commercially available at this time. A certain amount of "drag" is inherent in such a system, even when lubricated glass syringes are used. A new type of hydraulic pump without moving parts and with less inherent drag has been put on the market.[11] This low compliance system gives accurate recording of peristaltic pressure at low infusion rates of 0.6 ml/min or less.

OTHER VARIABLES AFFECTING PRESSURE RECORDINGS

Other variables not specifically related to infusion systems include (1) spatial variables, (2) respiratory variation, (3) artefacts, (4) type of swallow, (5) intra- and interobserver variables, and (6) the effect of drugs, hormones, and emotional factors.

1. Spatial Variables. Recent studies have shown that both upper and lower sphincter pressure profiles are not axially symmetrical.[12, 13] Different pressures are exerted in different quadrants. The reasons for

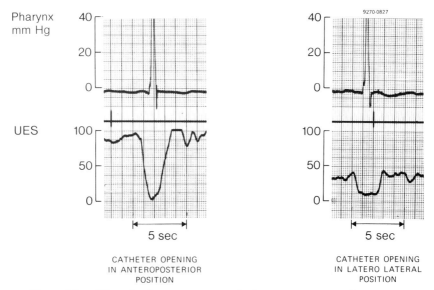

Figure 4-5. Effect of catheter position on the UES pressure recording in the same patient. Rotation of the catheter from an anteroposterior to a lateral position results in a reduction of resting and postdeglutitive pressures.

this are not totally understood, but the phenomenon is probably related to extraluminal anatomic differences. Pressures in the upper esophageal sphincter (UES) show the greatest spatial variability, with a markedly increased pressure in the anteroposterior direction compared with the lateral direction. Figure 4–5 demonstrates the effect on UES pressure produced by rotation of the catheter assembly 45 degrees. Differences in the LES are present to a lesser degree, with the greatest pressure exerted in the left lateral axis. It is not usually possible to know the spatial orientation of the catheter openings. Construction of catheter assemblies does vary, with three or four catheter openings usually oriented at 90 to 120 degrees to each other.

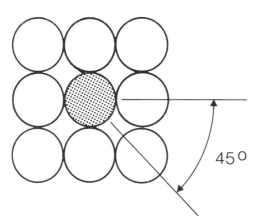

Figure 4-6. Eight-lumen catheter assembly. Spatial differences in sphincter pressure can be better assessed with this unit.

Eight-lumen catheter assemblies have been developed for special research studies, with openings 45 degrees apart (Fig. 4–6). Studies using the 8-lumen assembly can better document the spatial differences in sphincter pressure, but they are not generally practical for clinical studies. When three or four lumen assemblies are used, differences in sphincter pressure may be present from catheter to catheter. Under these circumstances, any determination of "true" sphincter pressure will simply be an estimate, usually the result of averaging pressures from all catheters. Obviously, the more sphincter pressures that are obtained, the better the approximation of true sphincter pressure. Obtaining only one interpretable reading through the UES (which may often happen) will obviously result in inaccurate sphincter pressure measurement. Pope[14] has recently commented on the difficulties of arriving at valid sphincter pressure measurements.

2. *Respiratory Variation.* Respiratory effect on intraluminal pressure is easily appreciated on manometric tracings. Inspiration increases intragastric pressure and decreases intraesophageal pressure. Changes are of the order of 2 to 5 mm Hg in the stomach and 2 to 10 mm Hg in the esophagus, depending on the depth of respiration. Determination of sphincter pressure may be significantly affected by respiratory variation. End-expiratory pressures are usually used in determining LESP, but mid-respiratory or end-inspiratory pressure could be used (Fig. 4–7). The rationale for using end-expiratory pressures is that (1) there is less variation in the measurement with depth of respiration, and (2) the end-expiratory pressure is the lowest sphincter pressure exerted during the respiratory cycle, giving a minimal estimate of sphincter "barrier" to reflux. The values for sphincter pressure in a given laboratory will depend on which measurement is used.

Use of a rapid pull-though technique (RPT) may resolve this respiratory variable.[15] With this method, the patient is instructed to hold his breath in mid-respiratory cycle, and the catheter assembly is quickly pulled through the sphincter area, giving a sphincter profile not affected by respiration (Fig. 4–8). Sphincter pressures measured

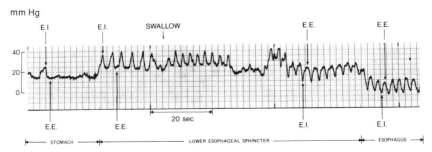

Figure 4-7. Relation of end-expiratory (*E.E.*) and end-inspiratory (*E.I.*) pressures during movement of the motility tube through the stomach, LES, and esophagus.

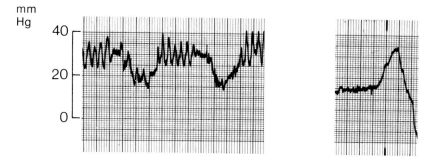

STATIONARY PULL-THROUGH   RAPID PULL-THROUGH

Figure 4-8. Comparison of the stationary pull-through *(SPT)* technique with the rapid pull-through *(RPT)* technique in measurements of LES pressure in the same patient.

by this method are usually greater than those measured by stationary pull-through (SPT). One may have to localize the sphincter by conventional SPT first, and care has to be exercised not to mistake artefactual pressure rises for the sphincter pressure when RPT is used. At times it is difficult to have the patient maintain mid-respiratory cycle during RPT without performing a Valsalva maneuver.

3. *Artefacts.* Any number of artefacts may occur during manometric studies that may affect the interpretation of tracings. Coughing, sneezing, gagging, retching, or yawning may occur and must be noted (Fig. 4–9). Repetitive swallowing caused by tube irritation may occur in some patients and may result in uninterpretable tracings, especially when one is attempting to measure resting sphincter pressure. Damping caused by less than optimal infusion speeds, air bubbles in the tubing, or plugging of a catheter with mucus is a common problem and must be recognized (Fig. 4–3). Realization that damping is occurring at the time of the study is necessary so that the infusion speed can be increased or so that catheters can be flushed. Artefactual disturbances must be noted on the tracing at the time they occur, since it is difficult to evaluate these changes at a later date.

4. *Dry vs. Wet Swallows.* Wet swallows in the distal half of the esophagus are of greater amplitude and duration when compared with dry swallows.[18] Wet swallows also result in a longer duration of LES relaxation. Interpretation of tracings requires knowledge as to which type of swallow is involved. Dry swallows are usually easier to use, but some patients have difficulty swallowing unless liquids are given.

5. *Intraobserver and Interobserver Variables.* There is significant intraobserver (two determinations made by the same observer) and interobserver (determinations made by two different observers) variation in the measurement of sphincter pressures.[17] Variability is minimal in the measurement of gastric and esophageal body pressures. Variation in reading sphincter pressure (UES and LES) proba-

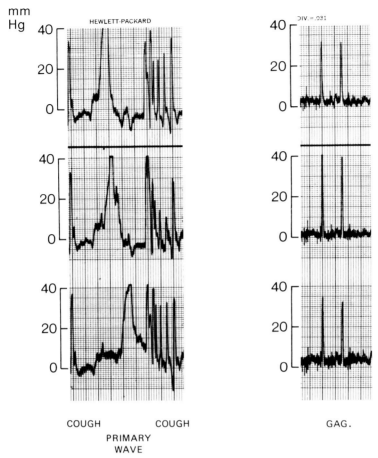

Figure 4-9. Artefacts influencing pressure recording. Coughing and gagging produce a simultaneous increase in pressure in all three leads.

bly relates to the judgment required in determining baseline pressure, eliminating effects of artefacts, and in interpreting return to base line sphincter pressure after deglutition. The determination of "resting" sphincter pressure may be difficult because of these factors. A wandering base line may make interpretation impossible. Failure to recognize that pressure has not equilibrated to a "resting" state following a swallow will certainly result in erroneous values. Averaging results of all resting sphincter tracings will minimize these variables. Double readings by the same observer and reading of the same tracing by two different observers will also reduce reader error.

6. *Drugs, Hormones, and Emotions.* The list of drugs, foods, hormones, and other substances that alter esophageal function continues to lengthen. A complete discussion of these factors will be found in Chapter 9. Emotional factors affect gastrointestinal function, and the esophagus is no exception. An extremely upset, hostile, or anxious

patient may demonstrate entirely different esophageal manometric findings than the same individual when studied in a more calm or relaxed state. Rubin[18] performed esophageal manometric studies in patients undergoing psychiatric interviews. An increase in nonpropulsive wave activity was demonstrated at times when affectively charged material was discussed. Care must be used in interpretation of esophageal motor abnormalities when the patient is disturbed at the time of the study.

REFERENCES

1. Kronecker H., Meltzer S. J.: Der Schlukmechanismus, seine Erregung und seine Hemmung. Arch. P.F. Physiol. Leipz. Suppl., 338–362, 1883.
2. Quigley J. B., Brody D. A.: A physiologic and clinical consideration of the pressures developed in the digestive tract. Am. J. Med., 13:397–406, 1959.
3. Pert J. H., Davidson M., Almy T. P., Sleisenger M. H.: Esophageal catheterization studies. I. Mechanism of swallowing in normal subjects with particular reference to the vestibule (esophagogastric sphincter). J. Clin. Invest., 38:397–406, 1959.
4. Winans C. S., Harris L. D.: Quantitation of lower esophageal sphincter competence. Gastroenterology, 52:773–778, 1967.
5. Pope C. E. 2nd: A dynamic test of sphincter strength; its application to the lower esophageal sphincter. Gastroenterology, 52:779–786, 1967.
6. Pope C. E. 2nd: Effect of infusion on force of closure measurements in the esophagus. Gastroenterology, 58:616–624, 1970.
7. Hollis J. B., Castell D. O.: Amplitude of esophageal peristalsis as determined by rapid infusion. Gastroenterology, 63:417–422, 1972.
8. Kaye M. D., Showalter J. P.: Measurement of pressure in the lower esophageal sphincter. The influence of catheter diameter. Am. J. Dig. Dis., 19:860–863, 1974.
9. Lydon S. B., Dodds W. J., Hogan W. J., Arndorfer R. C.: The effect of manometric assembly diameter on intraluminal esophageal pressure recording. Am. J. Dig. Dis., 20:968–970, 1975.
10. Stef J. J., Dodds W. J., Hogan W. J., Linehan J. H., Stewart E. T.: Intraluminal esophageal manometry: An analysis of variables affecting recording fidelity of peristaltic pressures. Gastroenterology, 67:221–230, 1974.
11. Arndorfer R. C., Stef J. J., Dodds W. J., Linehan J. H., Horan W. J.: Improved infusion system for intraluminal esophageal manometry. Gastroenterology, 73:23–37, 1977.
12. Kaye M. D., Showalter J. P.: Manometric configuration of the lower esophageal sphincter in normal human subjects. Gastroenterology, 61:213–223, 1971.
13. Winans C. S.: The pharyngoesophageal closure mechanism: A manometric study. Gastroenterology, 63:768–777, 1972.
14. Pope C. E. 2nd: Editorial: is LES enough? Gastroenterology, 71:328–329, 1976.
15. Dodds W. J., Hogan W. J., Steff J. J., Miller W. N., Lydon A. B., Arndorf R. C.: A rapid pull-through technique for measuring lower esophageal sphincter pressure. Gastroenterology, 68:437–443, 1975.
16. Dodd W. J., Hogan W. J., Reed D. P., Stewart E. T., Arndorfer R. C.: A comparison between primary peristalsis following wet and dry swallows. J. Appl. Physiol., 35:851–857, 1973.
17. Fox J. E., Vidins E. I., Bech I. T.: Observer variation in esophageal pressure assessment. Gastroenterology, 65:884–888, 1973.
18. Rubin J., Nagler R., Spiro H. M., Pilot M. L.: Measuring the effect of emotions on esophageal motility. Psychosom. Med., 24:170–176, 1962.

CHAPTER 5

THE PERFORMANCE OF THE ESOPHAGEAL MOTILITY STUDY

Techniques used in esophageal manometry may vary considerably, depending on the goals of the study. Under most circumstances, however, the technique used for the majority of clinical studies is fairly standard.

GOALS OF THE STUDY

It is of utmost importance to know why the manometric study is being performed and what particular information is desired. A careful history from the patient and any additional clinical information are extremely valuable in determining how the study will be performed and whether any modification of standard technique will be necessary. A thorough drug history, including use of alcohol and tobacco, should be elicited.

If the problem is one of gastroesophageal reflux, special attention to lower esophageal sphincter pressure (LESP) recording will be necessary. In addition, intraluminal pH studies and a Bernstein test will have to be considered. Disorders of the pharynx, UES, and upper esophagus may require a different approach and may pose certain technical difficulties. In certain motor disorders, alteration of infusion speeds may be required when the body of the esophagus is studied.

TYPES OF CATHETER ASSEMBLY

Most manometric studies of the esophagus are now performed using three perfused open-tipped catheters. Distal side openings are made 5 cm apart and with approximately 120 degrees between adja-

41

TABLE 5-1. *Procedural Checklist for Performing*
Esophageal Motility Study

1. Instruct patient to fast.
2. Direct patient to discontinue drugs, tobacco, and alcohol.
3. Check equipment.
4. Calibrate recorder.
5. Adjust zero base line on all channels.
6. Inform and reassure patient about procedure.
7. Insert catheter assembly.
8. Attach respiration and swallowing belts.
9. If pH studies are to be done, calibrate pH and place reference electrode.
10. Flush bubbles out of system.
11. Record base line gastric pressures.
12. Perform pull-through study of LES.
13. Perform esophageal body study with swallows.
14. Perform pull-through study of UES.

cent openings. A fourth catheter may be added for acid perfusion studies (see later discussion). An intraesophageal pH electrode may also be glued to the assembly if desired (see later discussion). For special studies, catheter openings may be at the same level (to give simultaneous readings of sphincter pressure in different quadrants) or at 1 to 2 cm intervals if desired. Many laboratories have several different assemblies available so that they are able to modify techniques depending on the clinical situation.

PROCEDURE*

The patient is instructed to fast for the procedure, usually from the night before. Drugs known to affect esophageal function, such as anticholinergics, should be discontinued prior to the study. Tobacco and alcohol should also be withheld prior to the examination.

The equipment used should be carefully checked prior to starting the examination. Tubing must be flushed of all air bubbles and should be inspected for any debris that might plug it. If water-filled strain gauges are used, they also should be cleared of any small bubbles that might be present. The infusion pump should be functioning correctly, and the appropriate infusion rate should be selected. Only glass syringes should be used, and these should be frequently greased to eliminate system "drag." Stopcock leaks must be eliminated. If a hydraulic capillary infusion system is used, selection of hydraulic pressure will determine infusion rate. Air bubbles can be avoided by using boiled distilled water.

Calibration of the recorder is now necessary. Pressures are commonly recorded in mm Hg, although cm H_2O may also be used.

---

*See Table 5-1.

Calibration of each channel using a blood pressure manometer is easily accomplished. Calibration of pressure may not be necessary every time the machine is used; this will depend on the recorder used. Some newer recorders may be internally calibrated. Calibration may be affected by very rapid infusion speeds; with lower infusion speeds, little effect on calibration of zero base line has been noted.

Base line zero atmospheric pressure must be adjusted on all the channels recording pressure. This is done by placing the transducers, water-filled and open to air, at a height approximate to that of the midaxillary line of the patient while in the supine position. In patients with severe kyphoscoliosis or increased anteroposterior diameter (as in emphysema), it may be difficult to estimate the level of the esophagus.

After the patient has been interviewed and a careful history obtained, the exact nature of the procedure is explained. The patient should be informed of the possible discomfort of the procedure and of the tendency to gag and retch. Reassurance must be given that the operator will be gentle and not cause pain. Patients generally have great fear of gagging, of not being able to breathe with the tube in place, or of being unable to swallow the tubing at all. It is helpful to inform the patient that a certain amount of gagging is commonly experienced by all patients. If care is taken to allay the patient's fears prior to the study, the patient's acceptance will be improved.

The catheter assembly is passed either through the nose (if the assembly is small enough) or through the mouth. Topical anesthesia for nose or throat may be used if necessary but is often not required. Most patients gag initially and require calm assistance from the operator. Passage of the assembly into the esophagus is best performed in the sitting position. A small swallow of water through a straw may be helpful in passing the tubing.

The catheter assembly is then passed further to a point at which all three distal openings are in the stomach, by prior estimation of esophageal length on the tubing. It may be necessary to disengage the catheter ends from the transducers to facilitate passage. When the patient is placed in the supine position, the tubing may be reattached to the transducers. Fluid must then be flushed through the whole catheter length (using the infusion pump) prior to initiating pressure recording. The patient must be made comfortable in the supine position (Fig. 5–1). At times a mouthpiece can be used that allows the patient to rest his teeth without biting the tubing. A mouthpiece is also helpful in keeping tubing stationary and minimizing movemen during the study.

If a record of swallowing or respiration is desired, separate belts around the patient's neck and waist may be used. Commercially manufactured equipment for these determinations is available and can be adapted to fit either one or two separate channels of the recorder. The

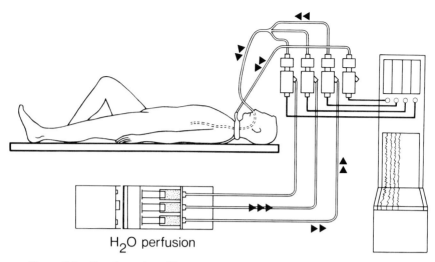

Figure 5-1.   Esophageal motility examination using a perfusion system. The patient is in the supine position. The pressure transducers are at midaxillary level and are positioned at the head of the patient. Water from the perfusion pump flows through the pressure sensors into the esophageal motility tubing.

number of channels available on a given recorder and the number of channels to be used for pressure measurement and pH determination will determine whether swallows and respiration can be monitored. Of the two, swallows are probably more important to record. If neither can be recorded, the patient can be observed for swallows and the paper marked at such times. This method is not satisfactory, however, since it is not always possible to observe the patient constantly, and since swallows may occur without being noticed. As it is imperative to know whether esophageal pressure responses occur after swallows, a swallow recording channel is necessary for accurate studies.

If intraesophageal pH is to be determined, both the intraesophageal electrode and a reference electrode must be used (see later discussion). A pH meter may be required, although some recorders have channels that record pH directly. Calibration of pH must also be performed prior to initiating the study.

After the tubing is flushed, the recording paper is started, and base line pressure is noted. The transducers should be positioned to be approximately at the level of the esophagus, and zero base line is then adjusted to the lower part of each recording channel. Recording from all three channels should demonstrate gastric pressure waves. If such is the case, all three channels will show identical respiratory excursions. Expiratory pressure will be 2 to 3 mm Hg above and inspiratory pressure 4 to 5 mm Hg above zero base line. Zero base line pressure may be calibrated to zero atmospheric pressure for greater accuracy if desired. If the catheter assembly has not been advanced adequately and if the proximal opening is situated in the esophagus, the proximal channel will demonstrate respiratory excursions that are out of phase with the other two channels. Confusion may occur in some instances, and there may be some difficulty in determining where catheter openings are located. In some patients with achalasia the tubing may curl up in the distal esophagus rather than go through the LES, causing difficulties in tracing interpretation.

When all three channel readings are in the stomach, the distance from the distal opening to the lower incisor teeth or to the nares is noted on the recording paper. The catheter assembly is then slowly withdrawn at 1 cm intervals, with distances being marked on the paper and recordings being observed at each 1 cm station. The LES is first recorded by the most proximal (upper) channel. LES recordings then follow on the next two channels at approximately 5 cm intervals. Should this sequence not be observed, the procedure must be stopped until an explanation is found and the matter corrected.

It is advisable to obtain resting LESP from all three channels at least once (instruct the patient not to swallow if possible as the LES is approached and traversed). More than one pressure recording from each channel is desirable, and the tubing can be reinserted and the pull-through repeated. Stationary pull-through (SPT) or rapid pull-through (RPT), or both, may be utilized, as previously described (Chapter 4). Demonstration of the LES with swallows should next be accomplished on all three channels if possible.

After the LES has been satisfactorily examined, the catheter assembly is pulled out at 1 to 2 cm intervals so that the body of the esophagus can be studied. During this part of the study, it is advisable to have the patient swallow one or more times at each level. If the patient has difficulty with dry swallows, wet swallows with a straw or syringe may be helpful. Such swallows should always be noted on the recording as wet swallows. Any artefacts such as retching, coughing, sneezing, or talking should be noted on the recording as they occur to avoid difficulties in subsequent interpretation. It is not unusual for such artefacts to be confused with nonpropulsive activity. It is important during this phase of the study to determine whether any of the esophageal pressure complexes are simultaneous (tertiary contractions).

If damping is present, infusion speed may be increased. If the magnitude of the esophageal swallowing complexes is very high, appropriate adjustment of pressure calibration on the recorder will be necessary.

Study of the upper esophageal sphincter (UES) is usually performed at the end of the procedure, since gagging occurs, which may cause premature termination of the procedure. Adjustment of water infusion speed may be necessary to avoid aspiration. In studying the UES, evaluation of coordination of UES relaxation with pharyngeal contraction is of great significance. Since events in the UES occur rapidly, it is helpful to increase paper speed for ease of interpretation. If possible, the UES should be seen on all three channels prior to removing the catheter assembly.

MODIFICATIONS IN PROCEDURE

Variable Catheter Assemblies.   The use of different catheter assemblies for special purposes has been previously mentioned. An 8-lumen assembly can be utilized for special study of sphincters, in order to eliminate spatial variability (see Chapter 4). If one does not have eight recording channels and transducers, a four channel machine may be used if first one-half of the recording is performed, followed by the other half after switching transducers.

Studies for Reflux.   Measurement of intraluminal pH is an objective and sensitive indicator of gastroesophageal reflux.[1] Although there is a general relationship between LESP and presence or absence of reflux,[2] measurement of LESP alone is not sufficient.[3] Presence or absence of reflux is best determined by measurement of intraesophageal pH.

An intraluminal glass pH electrode may be glued to the catheter assembly. A reference electrode must be placed in contact with a mucous membrane and is usually placed in contact with the buccal mucosa. Continuous pH recording is then achieved. The electrode tip is usually located at the level of the distal catheter opening so that pH readings are correlated with that manometric channel.

Gastric pH is determined when the catheter assembly is first passed into the stomach. Gastric pH may vary from 1 to 7, whereas esophageal pH is usually about 6 to 7. In order to test adequately for reflux, it is advisable to instill 200 to 300 cc of 0.1 N HCl into the stomach through the distal catheter before starting the pull-through. Under these circumstances, gastric pH will be 1 or 2. If reflux is not present, there should be a prompt rise to at least pH 6 as the LES is crossed (Fig. 5–2). Free reflux can be assumed to be present when the pH fails to rise above 4 as the LES is passed (Fig. 5–3). If the pH rises promptly as the LES is crossed, the electrode should then be pulled up to 4 to 5 cm above the LES. At this point reflux can be tested using either Valsalva or Müller maneuvers or by utilizing abdominal compression. If reflux occurs, a prompt drop in pH will be observed (Fig. 5–4). Spontaneous reflux without straining maneuvers may also be seen during continuous pH recording (Fig. 5–5).

Continuous recording of LESP or of esophageal pH may be utilized, since reflux is often not continuous but intermittent.[4] In such studies, elimination of catheter movement is important, particularly if continuous LESP is being recorded.

Acid Perfusion Studies.   The Bernstein test[5] can be modified for

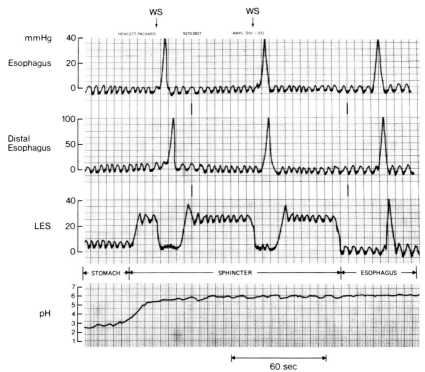

Figure 5-2. Absence of gastroesophageal reflux is demonstrated by a prompt rise in pH as the LES is traversed. (WS, wet swallow.)

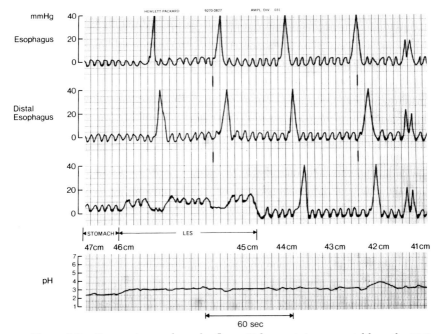

Figure 5-3. Free gastroesophageal reflux. pH does not rise appreciably as the LES is traversed. LES pressure is low.

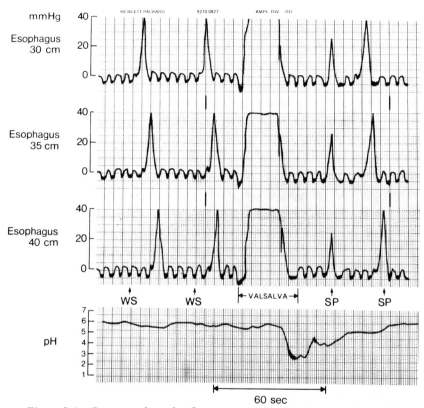

Figure 5-4. Gastroesophageal reflux occurs after a Valsalva maneuver. (WS, wet swallow; SP, spontaneous contraction.)

use at the time manometric studies are done. Simultaneous esophageal pressure recordings can be obtained as the acid perfusion test is performed. Bernstein tests are usually performed in the upright position, but must be done in the supine position if manometric tracings are being performed simultaneously. We have not observed that this slight modification of the test affects its validity. A positive test consists of exact reproduction of the patient's symptoms upon acid infusion and manometric findings of increased amplitude and duration of peristaltic waves, increase in nonpropulsive activity, and increased base line pressure when compared with the control period of saline infusion.[6] Figure 5–6 demonstrates an abnormal manometric response to acid perfusion in a patient with esophagitis.

COMMON ERRORS IN PROCEDURE

Performance of infusion manometry requires meticulous attention to detail. Mistakes in technique frequently occur and if unrecognized may result in incorrect interpretation of tracings (Table 5–2). Many of these procedural problems have already been discussed and are listed as follows:

   1. *Damping.* Damping may be caused by perfusion pump failure, empty syringes, air bubbles in the system, mucus plugs, inadequate perfusion (too slow a rate), leaks in the system, and sticking of syringes.

   2. *Errors in Measuring Sphincter Pressure.* These may be caused by:

   a. Not recognizing proper localization of a sphincter.
   b. Not recognizing spatial variation in sphincter pressure.
   c. Measuring "nonresting" sphincter pressure (persistent postdeglutitive elevated pressure).
   d. Too few sphincter pressure measurements to give a valid average value.
   e. Catheter movement during SPT measurement of LESP.
   f. Incorrect measurement because of a moving base line pressure.

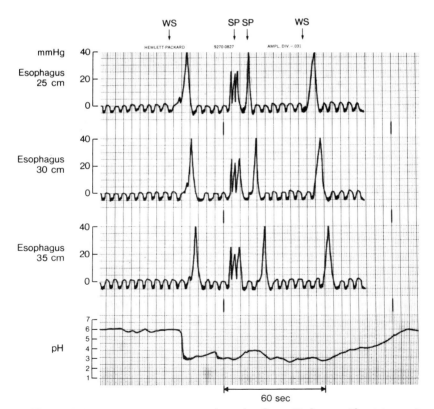

Figure 5-5. Spontaneous gastroesophageal reflux. pH drops without increasing intra-abdominal pressure. (*SP*, spontaneous contraction, *WS*, wet swallow).

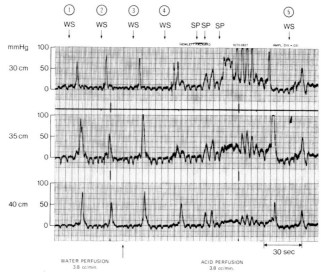

Figure 5-6. Motor response of the esophagus to acid perfusion in a patient with reflux esophagitis. Acid perfusion is initiated at the vertical arrow at the bottom of the figure. With acid perfusion, there is increased spontaneous activity (SP), base line pressure increases, a broad multiphasic wave is noted, and a nonperistaltic wave occurs after the final wet swallow (WS 5).

3. *Reversal of Recording Channels.* Incorrect hookup of the catheters to the transducers will reverse recorder readings.

4. *Artefacts.* Artefacts may be mistaken for nonpropulsive activity.

5. *Improper Calibration of Recorder.*

6. *Unrelaxed Patient.* Increased intra-abdominal pressure and straining will adversely affect the recording quality and may make the tracing uninterpretable.

7. *Incorrect Measurement of Catheter Length.* Incorrect catheter measurement may result in errors in determining the levels of the esophagus in question.

8. *Catheter Movement During Study.* Errors in catheter pressure measurement may result if the catheter moves during SPT.

TABLE 5–2. *Common Procedural Errors*

---

1. Damping
2. Errors in measuring sphincter pressure
3. Reversal of recording channels
4. Artefacts
5. Improper recorder calibration
6. Unrelaxed patient
7. Incorrect measurement of catheter length
8. Catheter movement
9. Errors in reflux testing

---

9. *Reflux Testing.*

    a. If gastric pH is greater than 4, reflux testing cannot be performed without instilling HCl into the stomach.

    b. Unless there is a volume of 200 cc in the stomach, little may reflux, even if the sphincter is incompetent. HCl should therefore always be instilled prior to testing for reflux.

    c. Retching during a Valsalva maneuver invalidates the test.

STANDARDIZATION

Because of the great variability in manometric equipment and techniques, there are no standard values for esophageal manometry. Values for sphincter pressure and peristaltic amplitude vary from laboratory to laboratory. Although desirable, it is unlikely that infusion manometry will be standardized enough to allow for such comparisons. When setting up a manometric laboratory, it is advisable to standardize equipment utilizing a constant diameter and length of tubing for all studies. Normal values for the laboratory can then be determined and used subsequently for comparison. As long as catheters and other equipment are not changed, then new normal values do not have to be determined.

If distal transducer systems come into general use, standardized techniques and normal values for esophageal manometry may be developed.

REFERENCES

1. Tuttle S. G., Bettarello A., Grossman M. I.: Esophageal acid perfusion test and a gastroesophageal reflux test in patients with esophagitis. Gastroenterology, 38:861–872, 1960.
2. Haddad J. K.: Relation of gastroesophageal reflux to yield sphincter pressures. Gastroenterology, 58:175–184, 1970.
3. Pope C. E. 2nd: Editorial: is LES enough? Gastroenterology, 71:328–329, 1976.
4. Johnson L. F., Demeester T. R.: Twenty-four hour monitoring of the distal esophagus — a quantitative measure of gastroesophageal reflux. Am. J. Gastroenterol., 63:325–332, 1974.
5. Bernstein L. M., Baker L. A.: A clinical test for esophagitis. Gastroenterology, 34:760–781, 1958.
6. Siegel C. I., Hendrix T. R.: Esophageal motor abnormalities induced by acid perfusion in patients with heartburn. J. Clin. Invest., 42:686–695, 1963.

CHAPTER 6

THE APPROACH TO · THE PATIENT WITH DISORDERED SWALLOWING

When a patient presents with a swallowing disorder a thorough clinical evaluation is mandatory. Failure to respect this dictum has led to unnecessary morbidity and mortality. Psychological factors should be considered only after the patient has had a completely negative medical evaluation.[1]

SYMPTOMATOLOGY

A variety of complaints will confront the clinician who is treating a patient with a swallowing problem (Table 6–1).[2] *Dysphagia* means "trouble with swallowing." This nonspecific term refers to a variety of symptoms including the sensation of food or liquid sticking in the esophagus, a gritty or scratchy sensation upon swallowing, and at times merely a feeling that "something isn't right" with the swallowing process. Dysphagia may result either from motor disturbances in esophageal function or from local anatomic lesions intrinsic to or compressing the esophageal lumen. As a general rule, motor disturbances produce episodic dysphagia that progresses slowly or is nonprogressive; liquids are swallowed with equal or greater difficulty than solids. Anatomic lesions produce relentless, progressive dysphagia, worse for solids than for semi-solids or liquids.[1]

Dysphagias can be classified on the basis of the location of the swallowing impairment (Table 6–2). *Oropharyngeal dysphagia* means "difficulty in moving the food bolus from the oral cavity to the cervical esophagus" (see Chapter 7). Symptoms include food sticking in the cervical region, pulmonary aspiration, and weight loss. Upper esophageal sphincter (UES) motor dysfunction is the usual cause, with an anatomic lesion being a less common cause. *Transport dysphagia* results when there is a problem in the passage of material through the esophageal body. Disorders of peristalsis (Chapter 8) may produce transport dysphagia. Luminal encroachment or extrinsic esophageal compression by benign or malignant disease can also lead to this form of dysphagia. *Esophagogastric dysphagia* results when there is impairment of bolus movement through the region of the lower esophageal sphincter (LES) into the gastric fundus. Symptoms in this area arise with either LES motor dysfunction or with benign and malignant obstructive processes.

Dysphagic symptoms are usually localized by the patient to the precise segment of esophagus involved. This is because the esophageal dermatomes are linearly represented on the anterior chest wall.

Occasionally, atypical patterns of dysphagia are noted (Table 6–3). Examples include oropharyngeal dysphagia resulting from gastroesophageal reflux or reflux symptoms referred to the suprasternal notch.[3] Dysphagia secondary to disordered peristalsis (e.g., symptomatic idiopathic diffuse esophageal spasm) may extend over much of the length of the sternum with radiation laterally.[4]

Esophageal obstruction usually occurs in patients who have had progressive dysphagia from an evolving benign or malignant stricture. On rare occasion, the process may occur suddenly without significant pre-existent symptoms. Esophageal obstruction may also occur in patients with severe esophagitis without stricture; in this instance, marked edema occludes the distal esophageal lumen. The patient with complete esophageal obstruction presents with total dysphagia, often with food impaction. Chest pain, odynophagia, and aspiration may also be present. Management involves immediate removal of the impacted food endoscopically or with digestive enzymes and then subsequent treatment of the predisposing condition.[5]

Inability to initiate swallows occurs with neuromuscular disease that impairs the voluntary preparation of food for swallowing. Parkinson's disease is the most common cause; patients with this disease have abnormalities of tongue and palatal movement that may lead to inadequate bolus formation.[6] Occasionally the inability to initiate swallows and to form a compact food bolus may be so severe as to compromise the patient's nutritional status.

Odynophagia, or pain on swallowing, occurs with a variety of structural and motility disturbances (Table 6–4). Neoplastic and inflammatory disease may invade the submucosal nerve plexus, leading to painful swallows. Esophageal cancer, retrograde extension of gastric cancer, and monilial esophagitis are common causes of odynophagia. Motility disturbances, usually manifested by very high pressure, nonperistaltic contractions, also cause odynophagia. Such high pressure waves may occur as the result of a primary motility disorder, or they may be consequent to esophageal obstruction.[2]

TABLE 6–1. *Symptoms of Esophageal Disease*

SYMPTOMS	DEFINITION	CLINICAL IMPLICATIONS
Dysphagia	Difficulty in swallowing.	Signifies organic disease. If relentless and progressive, suggests anatomic lesion. If episodic and nonprogressive, suggests motility disorder.
Obstruction	Inability to move food or liquid bolus beyond occluded esophageal segment.	Inflammatory or malignant occlusion of esophageal lumen.
Inability to initiate swallows	Patient unable to prepare oral bolus for transport.	Central nervous system disease, especially Parkinson's disease.
Odynophagia	Pain on swallowing.	Inflammatory or malignant invasion of submucosal nerve plexus vigorous simultaneous esophageal body contractions; obstruction.
Esophageal colic	Prostrating anterior chest pain, occasionally with swallows, triggered by certain stimuli.	Distinction from myocardial infarction or other cardiopulmonary catastrophe is difficult. Seen in symptomatic idiopathic diffuse esophageal spasm or in processes causing vigorous simultaneous esophageal body contractions.
Heartburn	Substernal burning sensation, usually with reclining or with processes increasing intra-abdominal pressure.	The symptom of gastroesophageal reflux. Implies a reduction in LES pressure, an alteration of normal esophagogastric anatomy, or an impairment of esophageal emptying.
Waterbrash	Presence of salty ("brackish") secretions in oral cavity.	Uncommon symptom of gastroesophageal reflux. Release of saline secretions by salivary glands in response to stimulus of reflux.

Regurgitation	Food or liquid ascending into oropharynx or nasopharynx after being swallowed.	Disease is usually localized to the region of the UES or LES. May be anatomic or motility disorder. Timing of regurgitation after the swallow important in determining level of lesion in esophagus.
Aspiration	Pulmonary soilage caused by spillage of esophageal or gastric contents into tracheobronchial tree.	Usually caused by disease in the region of the two sphincters. Fistula between esophagus and pulmonary tree also a cause. Acute or chronic lung disease may result.
Weight loss		May be caused by decreased caloric intake secondary to dysphagia or odynophagia. May also be consequent to catabolic effects of esophageal malignancy.
Gastrointestinal bleeding		May be brisk (hematemesis, hematochezia, shock) or occult (iron deficiency anemia). Common causes include esophagitis, esophageal ulcer, neoplasia, and varices.

TABLE 6–2. *Classification of Dysphagia*

TYPE	DEFINITION	EXAMPLES	
Oropharyngeal dysphagia (see Chapter 7)	Difficulty in moving food bolus from oral cavity to cervical esophagus.	Anatomic:	Intrinsic obstruction by malignancy. Extrinsic compression by thyromegaly or hypertrophy of cervical spine.
		Motor:	Oropharyngeal dysphagia caused by UES motility disturbance.
Transport dysphagia (see Chapter 8)	Difficulty in moving food bolus from region of UES to region of LES.	Anatomic:	Intrinsic obstruction by esophageal malignancy, benign stricture, Barrett's esophagus, leiomyoma. Extrinsic compression by cardiomegaly, tortuous aorta.
		Motor:	Achalasia, Chagas' disease, symptomatic idiopathic diffuse esophageal spasm, scleroderma, Raynaud's phenomenon.
Esophagogastric dysphagia (see Chapter 9)	Difficulty in moving food bolus from distal esophagus to stomach.	Anatomic:	Benign or malignant stricture, retrograde extension of gastric cancer.
		Motor:	LES hypotension, achalasia, syndromes with incomplete LES relaxation or incoordination with oncoming peristaltic wave.

TABLE 6–3. *Atypical Patterns of Dysphagia*

	CAUSE
Oropharyngeal dysphagia	Gastroesophageal reflux with or without distal esophageal stricture formation
Poor localization of dysphagia that extends over length of sternum	Achalasia Symptomatic idiopathic diffuse esophageal spasm
Gradual onset of dysphagia with poor esophageal emptying	Achalasia Proximal gastric obstruction ("gastric dysphagia")
Dysphagia following episode of heartburn	Disordered esophageal body contractions triggered by gastroesophageal reflux

TABLE 6-4. *Causes of Odynophagia*

CAUSE	PATHOGENESIS
Anatomic Lesion	
Inflammatory	
Severe reflux esophagitis	Invasion of submucosal nerve plexus
Monilial (candidal) esophagitis	
Caustic ingestion	
	and/or
Neoplastic	
Esophageal cancer	Secondary motility disturbance of esophageal
Retrograde extension of gastric cancer	peristalsis
Motor Disorder	
Primary	
"Vigorous" achalasia	Vigorous simultaneous esophageal body contractions
Symptomatic idiopathic diffuse esophageal spasm	
Incomplete LES relaxation or	
incoordination in combination with high	and/or
pressure esophageal body waves	
Secondary	
Vigorous esophageal body contractions	Incomplete LES relaxation/coordination
consequent to gastroesophageal reflux	
Complete esophageal obstruction	

Esophageal colic is a more prostrating form of esophageal pain. It may or may not occur with swallows. It is charactereized by severe, crushing bilateral anterior chest pain simulating the pain of myocardial infarction. Esophageal colic may be seen in a variety of circumstances but is usually associated with symptomatic diffuse esophageal spasm (see Chapter 8).

Heartburn is the symptom of gastroesophageal reflux. Substernal burning on reclining or with anterior flexion is characteristic. On occasion, a sour taste may occur as the result of gastric and duodenal contents reaching the oral cavity. Most authorities agree that gastroesophageal reflux results when the lower esophageal sphincter pressure (LESP) is low (<10 mm Hg). However, other intrinsic and extrinsic anatomic factors at the esophagogastric hiatus are also important in causing reflux. The severity of reflux symptoms is increased when normal secondary esophageal peristalsis is absent or impaired. Under these circumstances, inefficient "clearing" of refluxed material may result in intense discomfort and complications of esophagitis. On rare occasion, *waterbrash*, the release of salty secretions into the mouth, will accompany other symptoms of reflux. While the mechanism of waterbrash is unknown, it may represent secretion of sodium chloride and water by the salivary glands through an unidentified stimulus. The consequences of gastroesophageal reflux are shown in Table 6–5.[7, 8]

Regurgitation of swallowed material through the nares or oral cavity is usually the result of disease in the region of the two sphincters. Regurgitation immediately after swallowing suggests a structural or motor abnormality in the region of the upper esophageal sphincter. Oropharyngeal dysphagia, tumors of the hypopharynx and cervical esophagus, and Zenker's diverticulum are some of the lesions leading to immediate postdeglutitive regurgitation. By contrast, distal

TABLE 6–5. *Consequences of Gastroesophageal Reflux* [*]

SYMPTOMS
- Heartburn
- Dysphagia
- Odynophagia
- Regurgitation
- Waterbrash
- Acute and chronic pulmonary symptoms
- Overt and occult gastrointestinal bleeding
- Weight loss

COMPLICATIONS
- Bleeding esophagitis or esophageal ulcer
- Esophageal stricture
- Barrett's epithelium
- Pulmonary aspiration

[*]See Chapter 9.

TABLE 6–6. *Esophageal Lesions Causing Aspiration*

IMMEDIATE POSTDEGLUTITIVE
    Obstructing benign and malignant lesions of the pharyngoesophageal junction
    Oropharyngeal dysphagia secondary to UES motor dysfunction
    Fistula formation (congenital or acquired) between the esophagus and tracheobronchial tree

DELAYED POSTDEGLUTITIVE ASPIRATION
    Benign and malignant obstructing lesions of the distal esophagus
    Gastroesophageal reflux
    Achalasia
    Gastric outlet obstruction

ASPIRATION NOT RELATED TO SWALLOWING
    Nasogastric intubation
    Vomiting while in a semiobtunded condition

esophageal stricture, achalasia, and hypotensive LES may lead to regurgitation some time after swallowing has taken place. On occasion, the patient may be able to state whether or not the regurgitated contents are sweet or sour; this information helps to determine whether the food bolus has reached the stomach.

Aspiration may occur in varying degrees in patients with swallowing disorders. As pointed out by Henderson, "the precise effects of aspiration depend upon several variables: the quantity of the aspirate, the quality of the aspirate, the frequency of the aspiration and the response of the tracheobroncial tree and lung to the aspirate."[3] Of particular importance is the pH of the aspirated contents. Hydrochloric acid is extremely irritating to the tracheobroncial tree, and the patient will easily recognize even minute quantities of acidic aspirate. In contrast, patients with achlorhydria may not recognize the aspiration as readily, and pulmonary complications may develop without an obvious cause. On occasion, pulmonary soilage may be the only clue that esophageal disease exists. For this reason, unexplained pulmona-

TABLE 6–7. *Esophageal Causes of Weight Loss*

REDUCTION IN CALORIC INTAKE
    Dysphagia with impairment of normal bolus movement (anatomic lesion or motility disorder)
    Fear of swallowing:
        aspiration
        odynophagia
    Esophageal obstruction

CATABOLIC EFFECT
    Esophageal cancer

ry infection always demands an evaluation of esophageal function. Coughing after swallowing, nocturnal cough, recurrent pneumonia, and lung abscess may all occur as a consequence of esophageal disease. In addition, interstitial lung disease with impairment of diffusion capacity may result from chronic low-grade aspiration. In this condition, pulmonary symptoms predominate, and an esophageal basis may not be sought. The esophageal lesions responsible for aspiration are shown in Table 6–6.[9] The most common causes are anatomic or motor abnormalities in the region of the two sphincters. The evaluation of these disorders is discussed in Chapters 7 and 8. Tracheobronchoesophageal fistula is noteworthy in that very careful barium studies in multiple axial views are necessary, or the lesion may be missed.

Weight loss may accompany a variety of esophageal diseases. Its presence suggests lowered caloric consumption caused by motor or anatomic obstruction to bolus movement. On rarer occasions, odynophagia may lead to weight loss through fear of swallowing and decreased caloric intake. Finally, the catabolic effects of esophageal malignancy may cause weight loss independent of obstructive phenomenon (Table 6–7).

Gastrointestinal bleeding may occur in patients with esophageal disease. The bleeding may be brisk producing hematemesis, hematochezia, melena, and shock. Alternatively, blood loss may be gradual, the only clue being iron deficiency anemia. Reflux or candidal esophagitis, esophageal ulcer, neoplasia, and varices are some of the more important causes of upper gastrointestinal bleeding of esophageal origin. Some of these entities will be discussed in the ensuing chapters.

OTHER PROCESSES INFLUENCING ESOPHAGEAL FUNCTION

In approaching the patient with symptoms of swallowing dysfunction, the physician must be cognizant of systemic diseases that affect the esophagus secondarily (Table 6–8). Diseases involving the central and peripheral nervous system and both skeletal and smooth muscle may produce esophageal symptoms. Stroke, neuropathy (diabetic and alcoholic and mononeuritis multiplex), myasthenia gravis, myopathies, collagen vascular disease (especially scleroderma), and infectious processes may influence esophageal function and produce dysphagia. In these instances, the esophagus is an "innocent bystander" and is influenced according to the end organ damage produced by the systemic process.[10, 11, 12] At times, the major symptoms in these patients are not esophageal but are related to other major organ systems. For example, a patient with scleroderma and severe Ray-

TABLE 6–8. *Systemic Disease Causing Esophageal*
Dysfunction and Dysphagia

Central nervous system disease (especially vascular and demyelinating processes)

Peripheral neuropathy (alcoholism-associated, diabetic, idiopathic)

Myasthenia gravis

Skeletal myopathy (myositic, metabolic, muscular dystrophic)

Collagen vascular disease (scleroderma, systemic lupus erythematosus)

Raynaud's phenomenon

Infection (candidiasis, tuberculosis, herpes simplex)

naud's phenomenon may draw the clinician's attention to the ulcerated digits — the symptoms of gastroesophageal reflux may go unnoticed.

Disease contiguous to the esophagus may also produce significant esophageal symptoms (Table 6–9). Cervical spine disease, thyromegaly, recent neck surgery, esophageal irradiation, neoplastic mediastinal encroachment, and cardiomegaly may all produce significant dysphagia. Abdominal processes causing increased abdominal pressure may lead to symptoms of gastroesophageal reflux. Retrograde extension of gastric cancer may cause dysphagia and an "achalasia-like" syndrome.

Because systemic disease, as well as disease in the thorax and abdomen, can produce dysphagia and other esophageal symptoms, the physician must exclude these processes before assuming that a primary defect in esophageal function exists.[13]

Dietary habits, smoking, and medications may also influence esophageal function.[14, 15] Very hot or cold beverages may perturb normal

TABLE 6–9. *Contiguous Diseases Causing Esophageal*
Dysfunction and Dysphagia

DISEASE OF THE NECK AND THORAX
      Hyperostosis of the cervical spine
      Thyromegaly
      Neck surgery
      Esophageal irradiation
      Neoplastic or inflammatory disease of the mediastinum
      (e.g., lung cancer, tuberculosis)
      Cardiomegaly (especially enlarged left atrium)
      Tortuous aorta, aortic aneurysm, abnormal vessel

INTRA-ABDOMINAL DISEASE
      Increased intra-abdominal pressure aggravating gastro-
      esophageal reflux (e.g., neoplasm, obesity, ascites)
      Extension of intra-abdominal process into thorax (e.g.,
      pancreatic pseudocyst, retrograde extension of
      gastric cancer)

esophageal peristalsis and produce vigorous nonperistaltic contractions in patients with symptomatic idiopathic diffuse esophageal spasm. Dysphagia, odynophagia, and chest pain may result. Coffee, chocolate, and alcohol may lower LES pressure and aggravate gastroesophageal reflux. Smoking and anticholinergic drugs may do the same. Urecholine (bethanechol chloride), in contrast, increases LES pressure and is used therapeutically in some patients with symptoms of gastroesophageal reflux. A detailed summary of factors influencing LES function is given in Chapter 9.

PHYSICAL EXAMINATION

In most instances, the physical examination is not of diagnostic value in evaluating the patient with disordered swallowing. However, if the patient has esophageal symptoms, certain aspects of the examinaiton may be helpful (Table 6–10). As noted earlier, recent weight loss suggests neoplasia or some degree of esophageal obstruction to the food or liquid bolus. Halitosis occurs with stagnant retention of food as in achalasia, esophageal obstruction, and Zenker's diverticulum. A

TABLE 6–10. *Physical Findings Associated with Esophageal Disease*

Physical Finding	Significance
Evidence of weight loss	Dysphagia or odynophagia may be present; esophageal cancer
Halitosis	Stagnant food retention (e.g., Zenker's diverticulum, achalasia, esophageal obstruction)
Blood in stool	Esophagitis; esophageal ulcer; esophageal malignancy; bleeding esophageal varices
Lymphadenopathy	Esophageal cancer
Recurrent pulmonary infections; unexplained chronic lung disease	Aspiration of esophageal contents; fistula between esophagus and tracheobronchial tree
Neuromuscular disease; palatal speech	Oropharyngeal dysphagia
Spooning of finger nails and iron deficiency anemia	Cervical esophageal web (Plummer-Vinson syndrome)
Cervical "noise" with swallows	Zenker's diverticulum
Raynaud's phenomenon	Loss of normal esophageal body peristalsis; if patient has scleroderma, gastroesophageal reflux may be present

positive test for stool blood implies that esophageal malignancy, bleeding varices, esophagitis, or esophageal ulcer may be present. Supraclavicular or cervical adenopathy suggests esophageal cancer. Recurrent unexplained pulmonary infections or idiopathic chronic lung disease may be due to aspiration or fistulous transport of esophageal contents. Gastric bloating or borborygmus on inspiration is additional evidence for fistula formation between the esophagus and the tracheobronchial tree.

The presence of overt neuromuscular disease or palatal speech may help to explain the presence of oropharyngeal dysphagia. Spooning of the fingernails in a woman with iron deficiency anemia or pharyngeal dysphagia suggests Plummer-Vinson syndrome. Cervical "noise" with swallows is characteristic of a Zenker's diverticulum. Raynaud's phenomenon is associated with loss of normal esophageal peristalsis; in some patients with scleroderma, it may also coexist with a reduction in LES pressure and gastroesophageal reflux.

More often than not, however, the patient presenting with a swallowing problem will have entirely normal physical findings.

DIFFERENTIAL DIAGNOSIS

While dysphagia and odynophagia always indicate esophageal disease, other symptoms present problems in the differential diagnosis. *Esophageal colic* simulates the pain of myocardial infarction in its presentation, but can be differentiated by its relationship to swallowing, a normal cardiac examination, and a normal electrocardiogram. Esophageal manometry and esophageal barium studies may aid in the diagnosis[3, 16] (see Chapter 8). Other causes of chest pain such as dissecting thoracic aortic aneurysm, pneumothorax, pleural irritation, and rib cage trauma are usually differentiated by the clinical presentation and radiographic findings.

Heartburn may be coincident with, or aggravated by, other processes such as peptic ulcer disease, cholecystitis, hepatic inflammation, pregnancy, increased intra-abdominal pressure, salicylate ingestion, and anticholinergic therapy. A good history will include or exclude these other variables and aid in the diagnosis.

EVALUATION

A more definitive discussion of the evaluation and management of the dysphagias occurs in the following chapters. Nonetheless, a few comments on diagnosis are in order. *Oropharyngeal dysphagia* requires a thorough examination of the oropharynx, nasopharynx, and hypopharynx to exclude malignancy in these areas. In addition, cine esophagography rather than a standard barium meal is required in order to record the rapidly occurring swallowing events. Cine findings may be confirmed by manometric studies of the pharyngo-esophageal junction.[11] Finally, if a structural lesion of the cervical esophagus is suspected, rigid endoscopy with biopsy under direct vision is necessary.

Transport dysphagia requires an esophagogram and fiberoptic endoscopy to exclude structural lesions. Exfoliative or brush cytologies may be indicated if malignancy is suspected.[17] Esophageal manometry is indicated if the above studies are unfruitful. Studies to exclude cardiac disease may be necessary in patients with symptomatic idiopathic diffuse esophageal spasm.

Esophagogastric dysphagia is approached similarly to transport dysphagia. In addition to an esophagogram, a formal upper gastrointestinal series should be performed to rule out retrograde extension of a gastric carcinoma.[18] Special studies performed to evaluate gastroesophageal reflux are discussed in Chapter 9.

In general, the clinician should approach any patient with esophageal symptoms with the assumption that a structural lesion is present. Only after exclusion of such lesions, should one proceed to motility studies. Systemic diseases and contiguous diseases in the thorax and abdomen should also be excluded, since these may involve the esophagus secondarily.

Historically, structural defects in the esophagus tend to produce constant and progressive symptoms, while motility disorders cause intermittent nonprogressive symptoms. However, this generalization is frequently violated, emphasizing the need for a comprehensive examination.

REFERENCES

1. Phillips M. M., Hendrix T. R.: Dysphagia. Postgrad. Med., 50:81–86, 1971.
2. Edwards D. A. W.: Discriminatory value of symptoms in the differential diagnosis of dysphagia. Clinics in Gastroenterology, 5(1):49–57, 1976.
3. Henderson R. D.: Symptoms of hiatal hernia and gastroesophageal reflux. *In: Motor Disorders of the Esophagus*. The Williams & Wilkins Co., Baltimore, 1976, pp. 42–59.
4. Bennett J. R., Hendrix T. R.: Diffuse esophageal spasm. A disorder with more than one cause. Gastroenterology, 59:273–279, 1970.
5. Cavo J. W., Koops H. G., Gryboski R. A.: Use of enzymes for meat impactions in the esophagus. Laryngoscope, 87:630–631, 1977.
6. Donner M. W., Silberger M. L.: Cinefluorographic analysis of pharyngeal swallowing in neuromuscular disorders. Am. J. Med. Sci., 261:600–616, 1966.
7. Dodds W. J., Hogan, W. J., Miller W. N.: Reflux esophagitis. Am. J. Dig. Dis., 21:49–67, 1976.
8. Castell D. O.: The lower esophageal sphincter. Physiologic and clinical aspects. Ann. Int. Med., 83:390–401, 1975.
9. Belsey R.: The pulmonary complications of oesophageal disease. Brit. J. Dis. Chest, 54:342–348, 1960.
10. Fischer R. A., Ellison G. W., Thayer W. R., Spiro H. M., Glaser G. H.: Esophageal motility in neuromuscular disorders. Ann. Int. Med., 63:229–284, 1965.

11. Hurwitz A. L., Nelson J. A., Haddad J. K.: Oropharyngeal dysphagia. Manometric and cine esophagraphic findings. Am. J. Dig. Dis., 20:313–324, 1975.

12. Hurwitz A. L., Duranceau A., Postlethwait R. W.: Esophageal dysfunction and Raynaud's phenomenon in patients with scleroderma. Am. J. Dig. Dis., 21:601–606, 1976.

13. Earlam R.: Oesophageal abnormalities in various medical conditions. *In: Clinical Tests of Oesophageal Function.* Grune & Stratton, New York, 1976, pp. 265–306.

14. Pope C. E. 2nd: Physiology (of the esophagus). *In: Gastrointestinal Disease.* 2nd ed. (Sleisenger M. H., Fordtran J. S., eds.) W. B. Saunders Co., Philadelphia, 1978, pp. 504–511.

15. Pope C. E. 2nd: Motor disorders (of the esophagus). *In: Gastrointestinal Disease.* 2nd ed. (Sleisenger M. H., Fordtran J. S., eds.). W. B. Saunders Co., Philadelphia, 1978, pp. 513–537.

16. Brand D. L., Martin D., Pope C. E. 2nd: Esophageal manometrics in patients with angina-like chest pain. Am. J. Dig. Dis., 22:300–304, 1977.

17. MacDonald W. C., Brandborg L. L., Taniguchi L., and Rubin C. E.: Esophageal exfoliative cytology. A neglected procedure. Ann. Int. Med., 59:332–337, 1963.

18. Kolodny M., Schrader Z. R., Rubin W., Hockman R., Sleisenger M. H.: Esophageal achalasia probably due to gastric carcinoma. Ann. Int. Med., 69:569–573, 1968.

CHAPTER 7

OROPHARYNGEAL DYSPHAGIA

Oropharyngeal dysphagia is a symptom complex characterized by difficulty in propelling a food or liquid bolus from the oral cavity into the cervical esophagus. Patients with this disorder manifest a wide variety of complaints, including difficulty initiating swallows, local dysphagia or odynophagia, and symptoms of pulmonary aspiration.[1, 2, 3] Manifestations of associated neuromuscular disease are frequently present.

PATHOGENESIS

The basis for oropharyngeal dysphagia is not entirely known. Many neuromuscular diseases along the neuraxis are associated with this form of dysphagia. These disorders include central nervous system disease, peripheral neuropathy, motor end-plate disease, and skeletal myopathy.[1, 3, 4, 5] Neuromuscular disease is responsible for oropharyngeal dysphagia in 75 to 85 percent of cases (Table 7–1). Less frequently, local structural lesions in the oropharynx and hypopharynx are the cause (Table 7–2). Some patients have no associated neuromuscular or local structural abnormalities to explain their dysphagia. Despite the large number of diseases that can produce oropharyngeal dysphagia, it is usually caused by upper esophageal sphincter (UES) dysfunction. Abnormalities of UES relaxation or coordination are seen in the majority of patients with oropharyngeal dysphagia. These abnormalities may be detected by either cine esophagogram or esophageal motility studies and serve to separate these patients from controls without such symptoms.[3] These defects of UES function may be of two types: (1) failure of the UES to relax to cervical esophageal base line pressure and (2) failure of the UES relaxation phase to be coordinated with pharyngeal contraction. These two abnormalities may occur separately or together in any individual patient (Figs. 7–1, 7–2, 7–3, and Table 7–2).

67

TABLE 7–1. *Neuromuscular Causes of
Oropharyngeal Dysphagia*

CENTRAL NERVOUS SYSTEM
    Cerebrovascular accident
    Parkinson's disease
    Huntington's chorea
    Multiple sclerosis
    Amyotrophic lateral sclerosis
    Brain stem tumors (primary or metastatic)
    Tabes dorsalis
    Miscellaneous congenital and degenerative disorders of the central
    nervous system

PERIPHERAL NERVOUS SYSTEM
    Bulbar poliomyelitis
    Peripheral neuropathy (diabetic, mononeuritis multiplex)

MOTOR END-PLATE
    Myasthenia gravis

SKELETAL MUSCLE
    Inflammatory disease (polymyositis, dermatomyositis)
    Muscular dystrophy (myotonic, oculopharyngeal)
    Metabolic myopathy (thyrotoxicosis, hypothyroidism)

(Reprinted from Hurwitz A. L., Nelson J. A., Haddad J. K.: Oropharyngeal dysphagias. Am. J. Dig. Dis., 20:313–324, 1975. By permission of Plenum Publishing
Corporation, New York.)

    To date, no histopathological data on the UES in these neuromus-
cular diseases are available. Therefore anatomic-manometric correlations have not been made. Since the UES is composed of skeletal
muscle, diseases that affect the smooth muscle portion of the esophagus, such as scleroderma and achalasia, do not usually produce symptoms of oropharyngeal dysphagia. On occasion, however, a patient
with mixed connective tissue disease involving both smooth and skeletal muscle may have a motility disorder involving both the proximal
and distal esophagus.

    The most common neuromuscular cause of oropharyngeal dys-
phagia is central nervous system disease. Patients with Parkinson's
disease may have difficulty with the formation and preparation of the
food or liquid bolus.[6] Pulmonary aspiration and motor abnormalities
of UES function may be observed. One study did not find serious
dysphagia in parkinsonian patients, suggesting that patient selection
or other factors may be critical in the determination of symptoms.[7]
Cerebrovascular disease, especially cerebrovascular accident, is also a
common central nervous system cause of oropharyngeal dysphagia.

    Peripheral neuropathy may lead to severe oropharyngeal symp-
toms. Mononeuritis multiplex and diabetic neuropathy have produced
significant cervical dysphagia.[3]

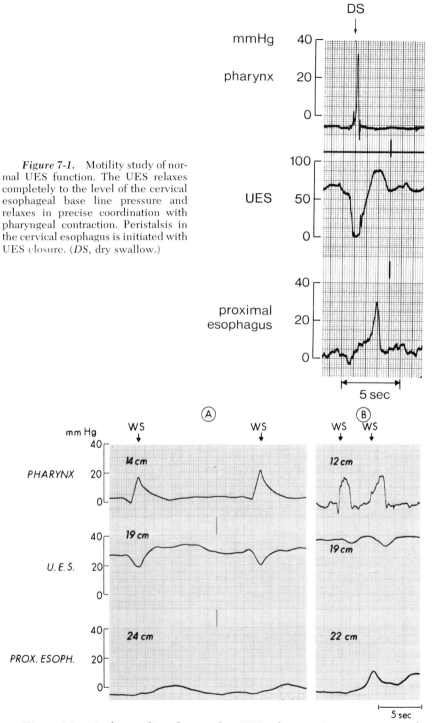

Figure 7-1. Motility study of normal UES function. The UES relaxes completely to the level of the cervical esophageal base line pressure and relaxes in precise coordination with pharyngeal contraction. Peristalsis in the cervical esophagus is initiated with UES closure. (*DS*, dry swallow.)

Figure 7-2. Motility studies of incomplete UES relaxation. In two patients with oropharyngeal dysphagia (*A* and *B*), the UES does not relax completely to the level of the cervical esophageal base line pressure. (*WS*, wet swallow.) Reprinted from Duranceau A., Jamieson G., Hurwitz A. L., Jones R. S., Postlethwait R. W.: Alteration in esophageal motility after laryngectomy. Am. J. Surg., 131:30–35, 1976 (by permission).

69

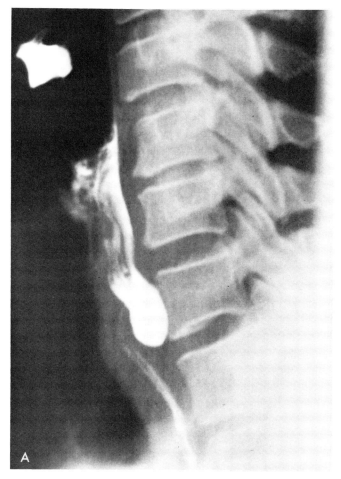

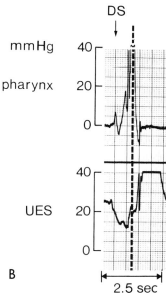

Figure 7-3. A, Pharyngoesophageal (Zenker's) diverticulum in a patient with severe oropharyngeal dysphagia. *B,* Motility study showing incoordination of the UES in a patient with a pharyngoesophageal diverticulum. The UES relaxation phase is not coordinated with pharyngeal contraction. Contraction of the pharynx occurs simultaneously with premature closure of the UES (illustrated by the vertical dashed line). (*DS,* dry swallow.) Resting pressure in the UES is low.

TABLE 7–2. *UES Motility Disturbances in*
Oropharyngeal Dysphagia°

INCOMPLETE UES RELAXATION: UES does not relax completely to cervical
                            esophageal base line pressure (Fig. 7–2).

INCOORDINATION OF UES WITH PHARYNX: Pharyngeal contraction and UES
                            relaxation phase are not coordinated. Most
                            common defect is the simultaneous contraction
                            of pharynx and UES (Fig. 7–3).

°The two motility disturbances may occur singly or in combination.

Myasthenia gravis, a disease of the skeletal motor end-plate, frequently presents with bulbar symptoms. Oropharyngeal dysphagia, especially with repeated swallowing efforts, may occur.[8]

Skeletal myopathies, including inflammatory disease of skeletal muscle (e.g., polymyositis), the muscular dystrophies, and the metabolic myopathies, may produce oropharyngeal dysphagia. Of particular interest is oculopharyngeal dystrophy, a disease frequently affecting families of French-Canadian descent. This disease is characterized by ptosis and dysphagia and progresses as the patient becomes older.[9, 10] Patients with oculopharyngeal dystrophy complain of inability to propel the food or liquid bolus from the oral cavity into the cervical esophagus, oral and nasal regurgitation, and frequent aspiration. Esophageal motility studies reveal low pharyngeal pressures, UES defects in both coordination and relaxation of the sphincter, and abnormalities in esophageal body peristalsis[11] (Fig. 7–4).

A large number of patients have oropharyngeal dysphagia for which no neuromuscular disease can be found. Included in this category are some patients with Zenker's diverticulum. Zenker's diverticulum may be associated with abnormal function of the UES. In particular, abnormal UES coordination with pharyngeal contraction and incomplete UES relaxation have been described[12] (Fig. 7–3B). These abnormalities of UES dysfunction are not seen in patients with Zenker's diverticulum. We and other observers have noted that many patients with Zenker's diverticula may have entirely normal motor function of the UES. This suggests that in some patients with this disorder the presence of the diverticulum need not signify a motor abnormality.

Local structural lesions may produce oropharyngeal dysphagia by either intrinsic or extrinsic compression of the pharyngoesophageal junction (Table 7–3). Oropharyngeal carcinoma, pharyngeal abscess, congenital webs of the proximal esophagus, and the Plummer-Vinson syndrome produce local dysphagia by intrinsic distortion of the solid or liquid bolus as it moves from the hypopharynx into the cervical esophagus. Extrinsic compression may occur with thyromegaly, senile

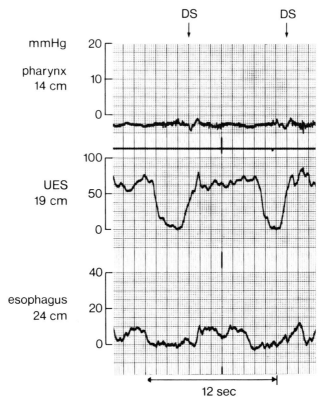

Figure 7-4. Motility study in a patient with oculopharyngeal muscular dystrophy. Pharyngeal contraction is absent, and swallowing is out of phase with UES relaxation (*DS*, dry swallow).

TABLE 7-3. *Structural Lesions Producing Oropharyngeal Dysphagia*°

INTRINSIC LESIONS OF PHARYNGOESOPHAGEAL JUNCTION
    Surgical resection of oropharynx
    Congenital webs of proximal esophagus
    Plummer-Vinson syndrome
    Zenker's diverticulum
    Inflammatory disease (pharyngitis, abscess)
    Oropharyngeal and hypopharyngeal carcinoma

EXTRINSIC COMPRESSION OF PHARYNGOESOPHAGEAL JUNCTION
    Thyromegaly
    Cervical lymphadenopathy
    Senile ankylosing hyperostosis of the cervical spine

°Reprinted from Hurwitz A. L., Nelson J. A., Haddad J. K.: Oropharyngeal dysphagia. Amer. J. Dig. Dis., 20:313–324, 1975. By permission of Plenum Publishing Corporation, New York.

TABLE 7-4. *Surgical Factors Causing Oropharyngeal Dysphagia*

Presurgical status of pharyngoesophageal junction and UES
Location and volume of resected tissue
Effects of muscle transection (laryngectomy, radical neck surgery)
Interruption of neural innervation of UES (sacrifice of the recurrent
    laryngeal nerve, disruption of the pharyngeal plexus of the vagus nerve)
Cicatricial scarring preventing normal laryngeal excursion (thyroid,
    parathyroid surgery; radical neck surgery; tracheostomy)
Adverse tissue effects of preoperative radiation therapy and chemotherapy

ankylosing hyperostosis of the cervical spine, or with cervical lymphadenopathy. Local structural lesions, intrinsic or extrinsic, are
usually diagnosed by an adequate physical examination and appropriate radiographic studies of the area. Since many of these structural
lesions are completely remediable, their presence should be excluded
before evaluating the patient for a motor disorder.

A unique group of patients presenting oropharyngeal dysphagia
are those who have undergone neck surgery or prior tracheostomy.
These patients may show a variety of motility defects resulting from
local scar formation, disruption of the neural and muscular structures
at the level of the UES, or perioperative irradiation for malignancy
(Table 7-4). Included in this group of patients are those who have
undergone radical neck surgery for carcinoma, patients who have had
thyroid or parathyroid surgery in whom the recurrent laryngeal nerve
has been sacrificed, and patients with tracheostomies performed for
respiratory distress. Postoperatively, cicatricial scarring may prevent
elevation and anterior rotation of the larynx with swallows.[13] This impairment of laryngeal excursion leads to weak pharyngeal contraction
and, as a consequence, to inadequate UES relaxation. Laryngectomy
patients not infrequently have postoperative dysphagia associated
with marked defects of UES relaxation and coordination.[14] Dysphagia
following thyroid and parathyroid surgery may result from interruption of the pharyngeal branches of the vagus innervating the UES or
from sectioning of the recurrent laryngeal nerve.[15]

CLINICAL MANIFESTATIONS*

Patients with oropharyngeal dysphagia will manifest a peculiar
type of swallowing difficulty, complaining that the food or liquid
bolus "sticks" or stops in the cervical region. At times severe pain on
swallowing may accompany the dysphagia, leaving the patient incapa-
citated for a period of 15 to 30 minutes. With the exception of the less
frequent structural lesions, the dysphagia and odynophagia subside,

*See Tables 7-5 and 7-6.

TABLE 7-5. *Symptoms of Oropharyngeal Dysphagia*

Food sticking in region of "Adam's apple"
Odynophagia in neck region
Nasal or oral regurgitation of liquid and food (immediately after swallowing)
Pulmonary symptoms (caused by aspiration)
    Immediate postdeglutitive cough
    Symptoms of acute pulmonary infection
    Symptoms of chronic lung disease
Symptoms caused by disease of central and peripheral nervous system (nasal speech,
    dysarthria, palatal sensory deficits, bulbar myasthenic or muscular weakness)
Complaint of weight loss caused by fear of swallowing
Occasional symptoms of gastroesophageal reflux*

*Gastroesophageal reflux may produce symptoms of oropharyngeal dysphagia.

permitting the patient to resume normal swallowing. Recurrent attacks of dysphagia or odynophagia are the rule, occurring at intervals of days, weeks, or even months. In addition to dysphagia, the patient may also note nasal or oral regurgitation of food and liquid. A common complaint is regurgitation of water or other liquids through the nares immediately after swallowing. Coughing immediately following swallowing suggests pulmonary aspiration resulting from anterior propulsion of food or liquid into the trachea. Such violent postdeglutitive coughing may be productive of recently swallowed food or liquid.

Patients with central nervous system disease such as amyotrophic lateral sclerosis or pseudobulbar palsy may complain of associated nasal speech and dysarthria. Weight loss is frequently a prominent complaint and is usually caused by inability to swallow an adequate amount of nutrients or by fear of swallowing because of pain or aspiration. Recurrent pulmonary soilage leading to multiple bouts of pneumonia, bronchitis or bronchiectasis may occur in patients with oropharyngeal dysphagia.[1, 2] As stated in Chapter 6, any patient with recurrent unexplained pulmonary infection should have an evaluation of esophageal function to assure that the esophagus is not a source of aspirated material.

Usually physical examination is not helpful in the evaluation of patients with oropharyngeal dysphagia. However, if the patient dem-

TABLE 7-6. *Physical Findings in Oropharyngeal Dysphagia*

Evidence of recent cerebrovascular accident
Presence of Parkinson's disease with tongue involvement
Brain stem disease involving cranial nerves IX, X, XI, XII
Presence of peripheral neuropathy
Myasthenic muscle weakness
Physical findings of muscular dystrophy or myositis
Laryngological evidence of obstructing lesion at base of tongue,
    pharynx, or hypopharynx
Surgical scar in neck
Thyromegaly
Cervical lymphadenopathy

onstrates manifestations of associated neuromuscular disease, physical examination may be very rewarding. In particular, evidence of recent cerebrovascular accident, Parkinson's disease, brain stem signs (especially involving cranial nerves IX, X, XI, and XII), myasthenic muscle weakness with repetitive activity, or evidence of inflammatory or dystrophic skeletal muscular disease can lead the clinician to a definitive diagnosis. Furthermore, the presence of a surgical scar in the neck, thyroid enlargement or enlarged cervical lymph nodes may explain the patient's dysphagia. A careful laryngological examination of all patients with oropharyngeal dysphagia is necessary to determine whether lesions at the base of the tongue or hypopharynx are present. The internist should not hesitate to obtain appropriate consultation if it is not possible to perform an adequate examination of the hypopharynx and larynx.

EVALUATION

The importance of an adequate history and physical examination has been emphasized in the paragraphs above. To document abnormalities of the pharynx, hypopharynx, and UES, however, the clinician must rely on radiographic and manometric studies. Conventional fluoroscopy and radiographic studies of the pharyngoesophageal junction are inadequate to delineate the rapidly occurring swallowing events that take place in this area. For this reason, in addition to the routine upper gastrointestinal series done on *all* patients with dysphagia, patients with oropharyngeal dysphagia should also have a cine esophagogram. Cine esophagographic studies are conventionally done at a speed of 30 to 60 frames/sec. The cine study may reveal abnormal movements of the tongue and soft palate, nonpropulsive pharyngeal contractions or asymmetric pharyngeal contractions, prominence of the posterior cricopharyngeal indentation on the barium column, inadequate UES relaxation, poor coordination of the UES relaxation with pharyngeal contraction, and evidence of pulmonary aspiration (Figs. 7–5 and 7–6). Thus, the cine study demonstrates structural abnormalities in this area as well as motor abnormalities of UES function.

Esophageal motility studies of the UES may be done with either perfused catheters or with transducers placed distally in the esophageal probe. The manometric abnormalities noted in patients with oropharyngeal dysphagia have been discussed earlier. To reiterate, the majority of patients will show either incomplete UES relaxation upon swallowing or failure of the UES relaxation phase to be coordinated with pharyngeal contraction or both. While not occurring in all patients with orpharyngeal dysphagia, these motility disturbances occur sufficiently often to explain the swallowing difficulty seen in these individuals.[3] Dodds and coworkers have commented on the

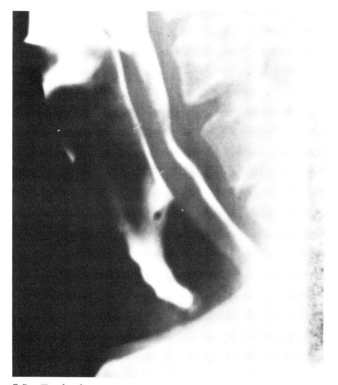

Figure 7-5. Tracheal aspiration in a patient with oropharyngeal dysphagia due to oculopharyngeal muscular dystrophy.

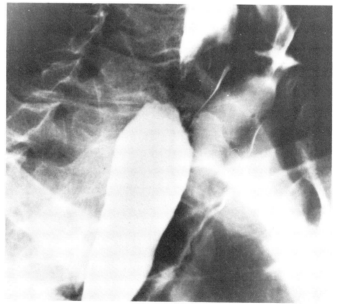

Figure 7-6. Segmentation of the barium column by abnormal motor function of the UES. A pseudotumor effect is created. Aspiration is present.

extreme difficulty of obtaining accurate measurements in the region of the UES.[16, 17] With improvement in measurement techniques using both perfused and distal transducer manometry systems, evaluation of the normal and diseased UES will be made easier.[18] Recently, the development of a glycerin-filled spatially-oriented manometry capsule has allowed for much more accurate measurements of the UES than previously possible.[19] The use of this instrument in evaluating patients with oropharyngeal dysphagia is yet to be evaluated but appears promising.

Nearly all patients with oropharyngeal dysphagia will have an abnormality noted on either the cine esophagogram or the esophageal motility study. In fact, most patients will demonstrate an abnormality on both studies. The cine and manometric correlation is good, although the esophageal manometry study is more sensitive in noting the presence of UES motor function.[3] This is because the cine esophagogram is a qualitative study and may not detect the full extent of UES relaxation nor the full degree of UES coordination with pharyngeal contraction. In addition, patients with oropharyngeal dysphagia may be hesitant to swallow an adequate bolus or barium, thus precluding adequate evaluation of this area. Nonetheless, we initiate our examination for oropharyngeal dysphagia by performing a cine esophagogram first in most cases. This may then be followed by esophageal motility studies if the cine esophagogram is nondiagnostic, or if further confirmatory data are required. In most instances, it is advisable to do both studies since different pieces of information are derived from each.

TREATMENT

Once the diagnosis of oropharyngeal dysphagia has been established and confirmed by appropriate studies, treatment can be initiated. While the management of UES dysfunction has been empiric and uncontrolled up to this time, the success of treatment has been good in selected patients. Three approaches are possible (Table 7–7).

TABLE 7–7.   *Treatment of Oropharyngeal Dysphagia*

TREATMENT	CONDITION
Medical	
L-dopa	Parkinson's disease
Cholinesterase inhibitors	Myasthenia gravis
Quinine, procainamide	Myotonic dystrophy
Treatment of thyrotoxicosis	Hyperthyroidism
Thyroid hormone replacement	Hypothyroidism
Corticosteroids	Polymyositis
UES Bougienage	Patients who have undergone surgical neck procedures leading to local cicatricial scarring
UES (Cricopharyngeal) Myotomy	Most patients with significant oropharyngeal dysphagia due to UES motor dysfunction

TREATMENT OF UNDERLYING DISEASE

The first approach is to treat any underlying medical illness that may be causing or predisposing the patient to oropharyngeal symptoms. Cotzias and his colleagues noted improvement in dysphagia in certain patients with parkinsonism treated with L-dopa.[6] As already stated, patients with myasthenia gravis often have significant bulbar symptomatology, including dysphagia. Treatment with cholinesterase inhibitors may improve the swallowing difficulty noted in these individuals.[8] Several types of skeletal myopathy may produce oropharyngeal dysphagia and may respond to medical management. The dysphagia of myotonic dystrophy classically is oropharyngeal in nature and may improve dramatically with the administration of quinine[20] or procainamide.[21] The skeletal myopathy of hyperthyroidism[20] or hypothyroidism may rarely present with oropharyngeal dysphagia, and in these instances management with appropriate agents has resulted in improvement or correction of dysphagia. Finally, patients with polymyositis who have difficulty with dysphagia and with the handling of oropharyngeal secretions may be helped by corticosteroid therapy.[22]

Although these medical conditions may respond to treatment with appropriate drugs, reports in the world literature are too scanty to make a definitive judgment about the role of medication in the treatment of oropharyngeal dysphagia. The use of medications in altering UES dysfunction is a poorly understood and untried field of clinical investigation. Pharmacological alteration of UES function is therefore an area greatly in need of research.

BOUGIENAGE

The second approach in the management of oropharyngeal dysphagia involves dilatation with mercury-filled bougies to alleviate the functional obstruction caused by the malfunctioning UES. Simple bougie dilatation of the UES may be efficacious in some patients, particularly those with previous neck surgery that has resulted in local cicatricial scarring. However, in most cases, bougienage does not have a long-term effect. Its use is contraindicated in patients with Zenker's diverticula because of the risk of perforation. The long-term effects of bougienage in dysphagic patients with neuromuscular disease needs further assessment.[9]

CRICOPHARYNGEAL (UES) MYOTOMY

The third approach to treatment of oropharyngeal dysphagia is surgical. Cricopharyngeal (UES) myotomy represents a major advance in the treatment of oropharyngeal dysphagia.[23] The rationale of this procedure is to decrease UES pressure or abolish the proximal high pressure zone by careful sectioning of the cricopharyngeus muscle. The procedure also involves sectioning 3 to 4 cm of adjacent cervical esophagus distal to the UES. This surgical approach remains extramucosal, which simplifies the operation as well as the postoperative course. The surgery may be performed under local anesthesia, which may be useful in seriously ill patients unable to tolerate a general anesthetic.[24]

Criteria for UES Myotomy

Extensive clinical experience confirms the fact that cricopharyngeal myotomy is effective treatment for oropharyngeal dysphagia.[3, 9, 25-32] Improvement of dysphagia, nutritional status, and pulmonary symptoms may be dramatic. However, despite the ease with which the procedure is performed and its low morbidity, it is essential that strict criteria for operative intervention be applied (Table 7–8). Myotomy should only be performed in patients having significant morbidity attributable to their dysphagia, such as odynophagia, significant sticking of food or liquid in the cervical region, marked weight loss, and symptoms or complications of pulmonary aspiration. In addition, confirmation of UES dysfunction by either cine esophagography or esophageal motility studies is a necessary requirement for operation, since absence of definable pathology suggests that another cause of the dysphagia must be sought. Finally, patients with significant gastroesophageal reflux should not undergo cricopharyngeal myotomy, since they may be more prone to severe aspiration and regurgitation in the postoperative period. In addition, patients with gastroesophageal reflux may experience discomfort referred to the suprasternal notch and simulating UES dysfunction. Therefore, patients with oropharyngeal dysphagia in whom a complaint of reflux is found must have appropriate evaluation and treatment of the lower esophageal sphincter (LES) dysfunction. The theory that LES incompetence and reflux lead to UES motor dysfunction is not tenable based on present evidence.

TABLE 7–8. *Criteria for Cricopharyngeal Myotomy in*
Oropharyngeal Dysphagia°

1. Significant dysphagia leading to local discomfort, weight loss, or pulmonary soilage.
2. Confirmation of UES dysfunction by cine esophagography or esophageal motility study, or both.
3. Absence of clinically significant gastroesophageal reflux or gastroesophageal regurgitation.

°All criteria must be satisfied.

Results of UES Myotomy

More than 230 cricopharyngeal myotomies for oropharyngeal dysphagia have been reported in the world literature. Highly variable results have occurred in patients with central nervous system disease, including patients with vascular, degenerative, or demyelinating disease.[26, 30, 31] Patients in this category tend to have better results if voluntary tongue and pharyngeal movement is adequate, and if sensation in the oropharynx remains intact.

As in patients with underlying central nervous system disease, patients with a variety of peripheral neuropathies also have an unpredictable response to myotomy.

In contrast to patients whose neuromuscular disease is proximal to the UES, patients with primary dysfunction of the sphincter respond much more favorably to cricopharyngeal myotomy. Included in this group are patients with symptomatic pharyngoesophageal (Zenker's) diverticula and patients with oculopharyngeal dystrophy. Following cricopharyngeal myotomy in patients with Zenker's diverticula, an approximate 50 percent reduction in UES pressure occurs, while the underlying motility disturbance persists.[12] The results of UES myotomy in patients with Zenker's diverticula is nearly uniformly favorable.[25, 30] Diverticulectomy or diverticulopexy may be performed if the diverticulum is large or if ancillary symptoms related to the diverticulum itself (e.g., regurgitation) are present. Small diverticula may disappear spontaneously after cricopharyngeal myotomy.

While one would expect patients with oculopharyngeal dystrophy to have a poor response to myotomy because of weak pharyngeal contractions, in fact, most advanced cases of this disease respond very favorably to surgical intervention (see Chapter 10, p. 143).

In the patient who has undergone resective neck surgery, usually for associated malignancy, oropharyngeal dysphagia may arise for a variety of reasons, as discussed earlier. Some surgeons may perform cricopharyngeal myotomy at the time of major neck resections in an effort to alleviate dysphagia. In most instances, however, the surgeon will wait to see if the patient develops dysphagia postoperatively and will perform a myotomy at a later date if it is indicated. The results of cricopharyngeal myotomy in patients who have already undergone neck surgery are variable and depend upon the extent of the underlying pathology, the level at which the original surgery was performed, the amount of tissue removed at the time of the original surgery, and the adverse local tissue effects of radiation therapy.

A large number of patients with oropharyngeal dysphagia have no underlying disease to explain their symptoms. Because of the wide variety of patients in this category, it is not possible to determine whether the patient will benefit from cricopharyngeal myotomy. This is particularly the case since the underlying pathophysiology is not known in this relatively large group of patients. Nonetheless, surgical reports in the literature seem highly favorable in this group of individuals.[25, 26]

Complications Following UES Myotomy

While serious complications following cricopharyngeal myotomy are rare, sudden death and death from aspiration have been reported[26, 30, 31] and observed by us. Particular attention needs to be directed to the LES, since sectioning of the UES in a patient with an incompetent gastroesophageal junction may lead to massive tracheobronchial aspiration. For this reason, and because gastroesophageal reflux may contribute to the symptom of oropharyngeal dysphagia, great caution must be exercised in patients who have LES hypotension. Documented gastroesophageal reflux, gastroesophageal regurgitation, or severe distal esophagitis must be considered absolute contraindications to cricopharyngeal myotomy until the LES defect has been remedied (see earlier discussion). Bleeding at the operative site has only been reported in one patient and was readily controlled in that instance.[28] Other theoretical complications of cricopharyngeal myotomy, such as perforation of the esophagus, recurrent laryngeal nerve palsy, mediastinitis, aerophagia, esophageal breathing, and inadequate sectioning of the cricopharyngeus muscle, have not been reported.

Summary

In summary, cricopharyngeal myotomy is a major therapeutic advance in the management of patients with significant symptomatic oropharyngeal dysphagia. Good results, meaning improvement or disappearance of dysphagia, have been noted in 64 percent of all reported myotomies. Fair results, signifying some improvement in dysphagia but with persistence of bothersome symptoms, have occurred in 24 percent of operated patients. Only 12 percent of patients have been judged to have poor results, with either no improvement in dysphagia or deterioration in clinical status. Thus, with appropriate patient selection, the clinician can anticipate a favorable response to this procedure. Surgical failures are most frequently seen in patients with central nervous system disease, peripheral neuropathy, and in patients who have been poorly selected for this procedure (Table 7–9).

Careful follow-up of patients treated for oropharyngeal dysphagia should include assessment of dysphagia, sequential weights, follow-up chest x-ray, and repeat cine esophagogram. While esophageal motility studies are helpful for initial diagnosis and may be useful to assess the adequacy of surgery, manometric studies are not critical for follow-up management.[3]

Oropharyngeal dysphagia is not an uncommon clinical problem. The basis for this disorder is now being understood for the first time.[33]

TABLE 7–9. *Surgical Outcome of 230 Cricopharyngeal Myotomies Reported in the World Literature*

SURGICAL RESULT	PERCENT OF PATIENTS WITH RESULT	PATIENT GROUP WITH RESULT
Good: marked improvement or disappearance of dysphagia.	64	Most patients with disease localized to UES (Zenker's diverticula; muscular dystrophy)
Fair: some improvement in dysphagia, but with persistence of symptoms.	24	Patients with central and peripheral nervous system disease
Poor: no improvement in dysphagia or deterioration in clinical status.	12	Patients with central and peripheral nervous system disease

However, more effective management of patients with this disabling disorder will occur only if more rigorous clinical and basic research is performed in this field.

REFERENCES

1. Phillips M. D., Hendrix T. R.: Dysphagia. Postgrad. Med., 50:81–86, 1971.
2. Atkinson M., Kramer P., Wyman S. M., Inglefinger F. J.: The dynamics of swallowing. I. Normal pharyngeal mechanisms. J. Clin. Invest., 36:581–588, 1957.
3. Hurwitz A. L., Nelson J. A., Haddad J. K.: Oropharyngeal dysphagia. Manometric and cine-esophagraphic findings. Am. J. Dig. Dis., 20:313–324, 1975.
4. Donner M. W., Silberger M. L.: Cinefluorographic analysis of pharyngeal swallowing in neuromuscular disorders. Am. J. Med. Sci., 251:600–616, 1966.
5. Fischer R. A., Ellison G. W., Thayer W. R., Spiro H. M., Glasser G. H.: Esophageal motility in neuromuscular disorders. Ann. Int. Med., 63:229–284, 1965.
6. Cotzias G. C., Papavasiliou P. S., Gellene R.: Modification of Parkinsonism — Chronic treatment with L-dopa. N. Engl. J. Med., 280:337–345, 1969.
7. Calne D. B., Shaw D. G., Spiers A. S. K., Sterne G. M.: Swallowing in Parkinsonism. Br. J. Radiol., 43:456–457, 1970.
8. Murray J. P.: Deglutition in myasthenia gravis. Br. J. Radiol., 35:43–52, 1962.
9. Peterman A. F., Lillington G. A., Jamplis R. W.: Progressive muscular dystrophy with ptosis and dysphagia. Arch. Neurol., 10:38–41, 1964.
10. Victor M., Hayer R., Adams R. D.: Oculopharyngeal muscular dystrophy: A familial disease of late life characterized by dysphagia and progressive ptosis of the eyelids. N. Engl. J. Med., 267:1267–1272, 1962.
11. Bender M. J.: Esophageal manometry in oculopharyngeal dystrophy. Am. J. Gastroenterol., 65:215–221, 1976.
12. Ellis H. G., Schlegel J. F., Lynch V. P., Payne W. S.: Cricopharyngeal myotomy for pharyngo-esophageal diverticulum. Ann. Surg., 170:340–349, 1969.
13. Bonanno P. C.: Swallowing dysfunction after tracheostomy. Ann. Surg., 174:29–33, 1971.
14. Duranceau A., Jamieson G., Hurwitz A. L., Jones R. S., Postlethwait R. W.: Alteration in esophageal motility after laryngectomy. Am. J. Surg., 131:30–35, 1976.
15. Henderson R. D., Boszko A., van Nostrand S. W. P.: Pharyngo-esophageal dysphagia and recurrent laryngeal nerve palsy. J. Thorac. Cardiovasc. Surg., 68:507, 1974.
16. Dodds W. J., Steward E. T., Hogan W. J., Stef J. J., Arndorfer R. C.: Effect of esophageal movement on intraluminal esophageal pressure recording. Gastroenterology, 67:592–600, 1974.
17. Dodds W. J., Stef J. J., Hogan W. J.: Factors determining pressure measurement accuracy by intraluminal esophageal manometry. Gastroenterology, 70:117–128, 1976.
18. Pope C. E. 2nd, Christensen J., Harris L. D., Nelson T. S., Motlet N. K., Templeton F.: Diseases of the esophagus (work group I) In: A survey of opportunities and needs in research on digestive diseases. Gastroenterology, 69:1058–1070, 1975.
19. Welch R. W., Luckmann J.: The upper esophageal sphincter (UES) in man: Significance of radial asymmetry and precise measurement of closure strength. Gastroenterology, 72:1168, 1977.
20. Leach W.: Generalized muscular weakness presenting as pharyngeal dysphagia. J. Laryngol. Otol., 76:237–240, 1962.
21. Casey E. B.: Dystrophica myotonica presenting with dysphagia. Br. Med. J., 2:443, 1971.
22. Vignos P. J., Bowling G. G., Eatkins M. P.: Polymyositis; Effect of corticosteroids on final result. Arch. Intern. Med., 114:263–277, 1964.
23. Ellis F. H.: Upper esophageal sphincter in health and disease. Surg. Clin. North Am., 51:533–565, 1971.

24. Hiebert C. A.: Surgery for cricopharyngeal dysfunction under local anesthesia. Am. J. Surg., 131:423–427, 1976.
25. Sutherland H. D.: Cricopharyngeal achalasia. J. Thorac. Cardiovasc. Surg., 43:114–126, 1962.
26. Blakeley W. R., Garety E. J., Smith D. E.: Section of the cricopharyngeus muscle for dysphagia. Arch. Surg., 96:745–762, 1968.
27. Montgomery W. W., Lynch J. P.: Oculopharyngeal muscular dystrophy treated by inferior constrictor myotomy. Trans. Am. Acad. Ophthalmol. Otolaryngol., 75:986–993, 1971.
28. Mladick R. A., Horton C. F., Adamsen J. E.: Cricopharyngeal myotomy. Arch. Surg., 102:1–5, 1971.
29. Mills C. P.: Dysphagia in pharyngeal paralysis treated by cricopharyngeal myotomy. Lancet, 1:455–457, 1973.
30. Akl B. F., Blakeley W. R.: Late assessment of results of cricopharyngeal myotomy for cervical dysphagia. Am. J. Surg., 128:818–822, 1974.
31. Mitchell R. L., Armanini G. B.: Cricopharyngeal myotomy. Treatment of dysphagia. Ann. Surg., 181:262–266, 1975.
32. Hurwitz A. L., Duranceau A.: Upper esophageal sphincter dysfunction: Pathogenesis and treatment. Am. J. Dig. Dis., 23:275–281, 1978.
33. Palmer E. D.: Disorders of the cricopharyngeus muscle: A review. Gastroenterology, 71:510–519, 1976.

CHAPTER 8

DISORDERS OF ESOPHAGEAL PERISTALSIS

INTRODUCTION

The mechanisms mediating normal esophageal peristalsis remain obscure.[1] The physiology of normal peristalsis is discussed in Chapter 3. Disorders of esophageal peristalsis occur when perturbations in the normal control mechanisms result in abnormalities of wave velocity and wave pressure. Most diseases influencing esophageal peristalsis result in a marked reduction in the percent of swallows that are followed by normal propagative waves. In addition, many of these diseases will result in reduction or amplification of the esophageal wave pressure.

In most instances, the loss of esophageal peristalsis does not result in symptoms unless confounding motor abnormalities are also present. This is because the human esophagus is capable of emptying by gravity whether or not peristalsis is present. However, symptoms will result if the esophageal body waves are of very high pressure or if LES dysfunction exists. In the former situation, very high pressure nonperistaltic esophageal waves may cause dysphagia or pain owing to marked impairment of bolus propagation and irritation of sensory nerves in the esophageal wall. In the latter situation, LES hypotension may lead to symptoms of gastroesophageal reflux or stricture formation, while incomplete LES relaxation will result in poor esophageal emptying with its attendant complications.

This chapter will deal with the three major diseases of esophageal peristalsis: achalasia, symptomatic idiopathic diffuse esophageal spasm (SIDES), and esophageal scleroderma. In addition, other diseases or syndromes known to influence esophageal peristalsis will be discussed.

85

ACHALASIA

Achalasia is rare. Its worldwide incidence is 1 in every 100,000 people.[2] It affects both sexes equally and has no racial predilection. Despite its rarity, achalasia is an important disease because it represents a model of disordered peristalsis and of LES dysfunction.

PATHOGENESIS

The basis for the deranged motor activity in achalasia remains unexplained. Epidemiologic studies have failed to reveal hereditary influences, although a few cases have been described in siblings.[3]

Microscopic studies of the esophagus in achalasia reveal loss of ganglion cells in Auerbach's plexus, which is situated between the inner circular and outer longitudinal muscle layers. These intrinsic motor neurons are either reduced in number or entirely absent.[4, 5] This abnormality may exist in all levels of the striated and smooth muscled esophagus, but it is most prominent in the distal portion, including the LES. In addition to showing this loss of ganglion cells, light and electron microscopy have revealed nonspecific changes in smooth muscle, including sclerosis of muscle and loss of the intermuscular connections called nexuses. Histopathologic changes also exist in the preganglionic nerve axons and in their brainstem nuclei.[4] Present evidence suggests that the axonal and brainstem nuclear changes are the result of retrograde degeneration, the primary process being loss of the esophageal wall ganglionic plexus. The basis for the myoneural changes in achalasia is totally obscure.

Chagas' disease produces a motor disturbance in esophageal function indistinguishable from classic achalasia. Chagas' disease is endemic to South America, especially in certain parts of Brazil, and is caused by infection with *Trypanosoma cruzi*. Chagas' disease will also cause dilatation and motor dysfunction of the duodenum, colon, rectum, and ureter. A chagasic megaesophagus represents an "experiment of nature," in which the toxic effects of the parasite lead to denervation of the esophagus.[6]

The motor findings in achalasia include:

1. normal functioning of the UES,
2. absence of normal esophageal peristalsis,
3. a hypertensive LES,
4. incomplete LES relaxation with swallows, and
5. hypersensitivity of the smooth muscle esophagus to extrinsic cholinergic stimulation.[7]

While the derangements in esophageal body peristalsis reflect the damage to the ganglionic plexus in achalasia, the abnormalities of

LES function are not intuitively obvious. Cohen, Lipshutz, and Hughes proposed that the lower esophageal sphincter hypertension in achalasia was due to supersensitivity of the sphincter to gastrin.[8] Dose-response curves indicated that this supersensitivity to intravenous boluses of gastrin I persisted after treatment of the achalasia by pneumatic dilatation. However, these observations were made using pharmacologic doses of gastrin I, and the relevance of these data to the pathophysiology of LES dysfunction in achalasia is yet to be determined. An alternative explanation for the LES abnormality would be some loss of the inhibitory impulses that maintain the resting tone of the LES, leading to an increased LES resting pressure. In addition, reduction of the peripheral activity of the vagus nerve might explain the incomplete relaxation of the LES, since it is speculated that LES relaxation is mediated by special noncholinergic, nonadrenergic fibers carried in the peripheral vagus nerve.[9]

For the present, however, explanations for the peristaltic and LES abnormalities of achalasia remain speculative.

CLINICAL MANIFESTATIONS*

The majority of patients with achalasia first seek medical attention between the ages of 35 and 45 years, although small children and the elderly may also have symptoms.[5] The principal symptom in achalasia is dysphagia. Patients are conscious that food and liquid do not easily pass the region of the lower esophageal sphincter and point to this area at the level of the xiphoid process in describing their complaint. The degree of dysphagia is highly variable in different patients, being severe in some and subtle in others. Some patients may be asymptomatic, recognizing their dysphagia only in retrospect, after treatment of the disease. Some individuals will complain of

---

*See Table 8–1.

TABLE 8–1.   *Clinical Manifestations of Achalasia*

Dysphagia
Odynophagia or esophageal colic (seen in "vigorous" achalasia)
Weight loss
Halitosis
Pulmonary soilage
       Acute bronchitis, pneumonia, lung abscess
       Chronic interstitial lung disease of obscure etiology
Possible association of esophageal carcinoma
Gastrointestinal bleeding
       Esophagitis
       Esophageal ulcer
       Craniocaudad varices

odynophagia or symptoms of esophageal colic — these patients may have high pressure waves in the esophageal body, termed by some observers as "vigorous achalasia."[10] Weight loss consequent to the dysphagia may occur but is rarely severe since most patients are able to maintain a reasonable state of nutrition. Halitosis may be present, reflecting the presence of stagnant retained material in the dilated esophagus.

The most serious clinical complication of achalasia is tracheo-bronchopulmonary soilage through the regurgitation and aspiration of retained esophageal contents. In some patients, recurrent bouts of bronchitis or pneumonia may dominate the clinical picture, and the clinician may not consider an esophageal cause for these infections.[7] In fact, because there is usually little or no acid in the aspirated contents, the patient may not sense the usual irritation from aspirated hydrochloric acid. The subtle evolution of pulmonary changes in these patients may divert the physician's attention to chronic recurrent lung disease of an obscure etiology.

The association of esophageal carcinoma and achalasia is still unclear.[11, 12] Should cancer of the esophagus supervene, it usually does so in a patient who has had symptoms of achalasia for many years.[13] This possible association takes on greater significance because the radiographic and manometric picture of malignancy at the cardioesophageal junction can mimic classic achalasia.

Very infrequently, significant upper gastrointestinal bleeding may be observed in patients with achalasia. The cause of such bleeding is usually esophagitis or esophageal ulceration secondary to stasis changes. In rare instances, carcinoma in association with achalasia may cause significant upper tract bleeding. Craniocaudad varices, resulting from obstruction of the peri-esophageal venous plexus by the dilated esophagus, have been described as a cause of massive hemorrhage.[14]

EVALUATION

Clinical evaluation of the patient with achalasia involves radiologic, manometric, and endoscopic studies (see Tables 8–2, 8–3, and 8–4). A routine chest x-ray may reveal evidence of acute or chronic lung disease. In addition, the food- and air-filled esophagus may present radiographically as a prominent air-fluid level superior to and posterior to the cardiac silhouette. Finally, many patients will not have a gastric air bubble because of the combination of absent esophageal peristalsis and incomplete LES relaxation (Fig. 8–1).

Barium studies reveal varying degrees of esophageal dilatation depending on the severity and duration of the disease. Normal peristalsis is invariably absent. The nonperistaltic tertiary contractions are

TABLE 8–2. *Radiographic Features of Achalasia*

CHEST X-RAY
  Air-fluid level superior and posterior to cardiac silhouette
  Absence of gastric air bubble
  Acute or chronic lung disease
BARIUM STUDIES
  Varying degrees of esophageal dilatation
  Absence of normal esophageal peristalsis
  Narrowing in region of LES ("parrot-beak" deformity)
  Occasional presence of esophageal ulcer
  Occasional presence of epiphrenic diverticulum

TABLE 8–3. *Manometric Features of Achalasia*

UES
  Normal findings
ESOPHAGEAL BODY
  Resting pressure positive with respect to gastric pressure
  (pathognomonic when present)
  Precise duplication of wave forms in all channel leads
  throughout length of esophageal (pathognomonic)
  Complete absence of normal peristalsis (sine qua non for
  diagnosis)
  Spontaneous synchronous contraction occurring without
  swallows
  "Positive" response of esophageal body to extrinsic
  cholinergic stimuli
LES
  High resting pressure (usually >35 mm Hg above gastric
  pressure)
  Incomplete relaxation to gastric pressure with swallows

TABLE 8–4. *Endoscopic Features of Achalasia*

Dilated esophageal body without evident peristalsis
Ulcerated or inflamed esophageal mucosa
Presence of retained food and secretions in esophagus
LES tonically is contracted but will permit passage of endoscope
with only slight pressure
Coexistent esophageal carcinoma may occur in long-standing cases
Orifice of epiphrenic diverticulum may be seen

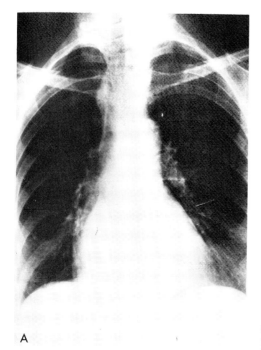

A

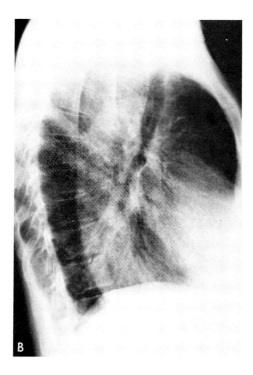

B

Figure 8-1.   Chest x-ray of a patient with achalasia. *A*, The posteroanterior view shows absence of the gastric air bubble and a double shadow along the right heart border. *B*, The lateral projection shows an abnormal fullness in the retrocardiac space. This constellation of findings is strongly suggestive of achalasia.

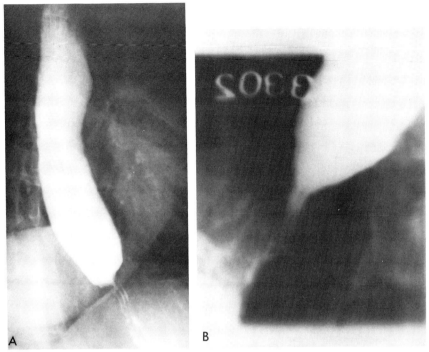

Figure 8-2. A, Esophagogram in achalasia. The esophagus is moderately dilated and tapers in its distal portion. B, Detailed view of the LES region in the same patient. Tapering of the gastroesophageal junction is seen.

best appreciated with the patient in the recumbent position, since an upright posture allows the esophagus to be emptied of the barium by gravity. The barium column narrows abruptly at the region of the LES in a configuration referred to as a "parrot beak" deformity (Fig. 8–2). While these x-ray changes are relatively specific for achalasia, they are by no means pathognomonic. Esophageal scleroderma with stricture or cancer of the cardia with retrograde extension into esophageal ganglia may produce a similar picture.

Esophageal motility studies should be performed on any patient suspected of having achalasia because the motility disturbances are diagnostic. The UES functions normally in achalasia (Fig. 8–3). The esophageal body shows multiple abnormalities (Fig. 8–4). Resting pressure may be positive with respect to gastric pressure. When this is true, it represents a pathognomonic finding not seen in any other motor disorder of the esophagus. A second pathognomonic feature is the precise duplication of wave forms in all channel leads. Complete absence of normal peristalsis is the sine qua non for achalasia, and the diagnosis cannot be made without this finding. There is one case report of restitution of normal esophageal body peristalsis in achalasia,[15] but this is an exceedingly rare finding. Spontaneous and syn-

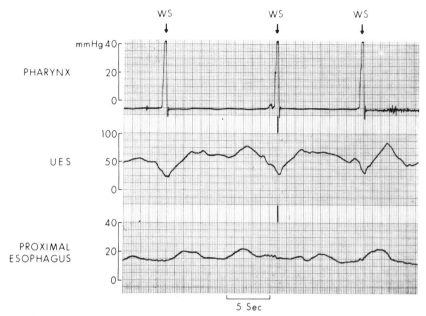

Figure 8-3. Motility study of the UES in achalasia. The UES is normal and relaxes completely to cervical esophageal base line pressure (10 cm Hg in this patient). The proximal esophagus has a positive resting pressure and contracts poorly with swallows. (WS, wet swallow.)

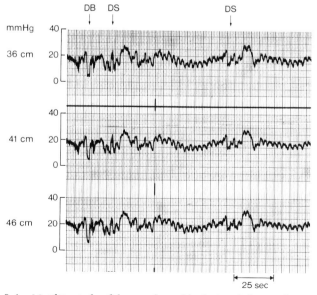

Figure 8-4. Motility study of the esophageal body in achalasia. Flat, nonperistaltic waves are seen with swallows. Wave contour is identical in all three channels. Resting esophageal body pressure is markedly positive. (DB, deep breath; DS, dry swallow.)

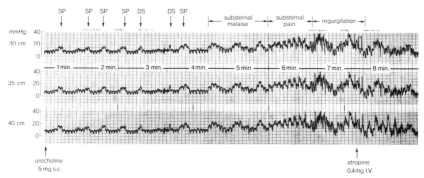

Figure 8-5. Positive esophageal body response to cholinergic stimulation in achalasia. Following subcutaneous administration of Urecholine, the esophagus shows a striking increase in spontaneous activity (*SP*). (*DS*, dry swallow.)

chronous contractions may be observed, occurring without swallows. When the patient swallows, simultaneous contractions occur, usually broad and of low amplitude. On occasion, particularly in the early stages of the disease, simultaneous contractions of high amplitude will follow swallowing.[10]

Because of local ganglionic denervation, the esophagus in achalasia follows Canonn's Law of "denervation hypersensitivity."[16] In the case of achalasia, the esophageal body and the LES hyperreact when an exogenous cholinergic stimulus is given to the patient. Either methacholine or Urecholine (bethanechol chloride) may be administered subcutaneously in very low doses. Shortly after administration of these agents, the esophageal body demonstrates an increase in base line pressure and a marked increase in spontaneous activity, with more frequent and higher pressure contractions (Fig. 8–5). Chest pain may occur following the administration of these cholinergic drugs; this pain, caused by esophageal spasm, can be relieved with intravenous atropine. However, if small 1.0 mg doses of methacholine or Urecholine are administered, patients will rarely have chest pain.

Manometric evaluation of the LES in achalasia shows it to be hypertensive, with resting pressures almost invariably exceeding 35 mm Hg above gastric pressure. In addition, while some degree of relaxation of the sphincter occurs with swallows, LES relaxation is incomplete[17] (Fig. 8–6).

Endoscopy should be performed in *all* patients with achalasia to exclude the possibility of coexistent esophageal cancer and to assure that the distal esophageal narrowing in achalasia is not caused by benign or malignant stricture. Endoscopy may reveal an esophagus inflamed or ulcerated due to stasis. The LES is usually closed but will permit easy passage of the endoscope following some minor resis-

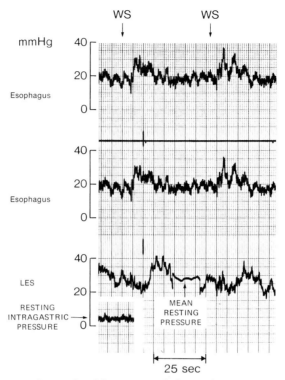

Figure 8-6. Motility study of the LES in achalasia. The LES resting pressure is at the upper limits of normal, and the LES relaxation to intragastric pressure is incomplete. Resting esophageal body pressure is markedly positive. (WS, wet swallow.)

tance. Biopsies and cytologic brushings of suspicious areas should be obtained.

TREATMENT

Treatment of achalasia is directed toward the hypertensive, nonrelaxing LES, since the peristaltic abnormality is almost always irreversible. Two therapeutic approaches are possible. One method is vigorous or brusque pneumatic dilatation of the LES. The other is surgical myotomy of the sphincter (modified Heller's myotomy). Pneumatic dilatation is an effective form of treatment for achalasia, especially in the early stages of the disease.[18] A variety of dilators are available. In this procedure, the bag dilator is fluoroscopically situated within the LES, and the bag is inflated to a pressure of 300 to 500 mm Hg, the end-point being full expansion of the sphincter zone during fluoroscopic monitoring. During the maintenance of high pressure inflation, the patient will complain of severe chest discomfort that eases after the procedure is completed. Upon its removal, the bag dilator may be covered with streaks of blood. The major complication of vigorous pneumatic dilatation is distal esophageal rupture or perforation requiring emergency thoracotomy. While such a complication is not common, it has been reported by some in as many as 5 percent of all dilatations.

An alternative treatment for achalasia is esophagomyotomy (modified Heller's myotomy).[19] This procedure is usually performed using a left transthoracic approach and involves sectioning of the longitudinal and circular layers of the esophagus from the most proximal portion of the gastric cardia and extending cephalad 7 to 10 cm into the more thick-walled portion of the distal esophagus. Postoperative complications include wound infection and the development of gastroesophageal reflux. The latter complication has led some surgeons to perform routine antireflux procedures following the esophagomyotomy.[20] Other surgeons, however, do not perform antireflux surgery unless significant reflux occurs in the postoperative period.

There continues to be considerable debate on the relative efficacy and morbidity of vigorous pneumatic dilatation versus esophagomyotomy in the treatment of achalasia. Data have been marshalled to support the use of dilatation as the first approach,[18] while contrary information suggests that esophagomyotomy is the procedure of choice.[21] Since all such studies either have been retrospective or have compared results at two different institutions, the controversy remains.

Several factors should influence the clinician as to which approach should be used. First, the local experience of the gastroenterologist in performing vigorous dilatation and of the surgeon in performing esophagomyotomy should be assessed. The percentage of successes and the number of complications for each procedure should be carefully weighed. Second, the stage of the disease is often a determining factor as to the choice of procedure. In early achalasia, in which the esophagus has not become excessively dilated or tortuous, either approach may be used. However, in advanced achalasia, in which a dilated, tortuous, "sigmoid" esophagus is present, vigorous dilatation may not be technically feasible, and a surgical approach may be preferable. Finally, a surgical approach is generally indicated in patients who have had prior unsuccessful dilatations.

Despite the controversy, the patient with achalasia can anticipate marked symptomatic relief when either vigorous dilatation or esophagomyotomy is properly performed. The degree of relief will be more marked if the diagnosis is made and treatment begun early in the course of the disease.

SYMPTOMATIC IDIOPATHIC DIFFUSE ESOPHAGEAL SPASM

Symptomatic idiopathic diffuse esophageal spasm (SIDES) is a syndrome in which chest pain or dysphagia or odynophagia is produced by repetitive high pressure simultaneous contractions in the smooth muscle portion of the esophagus.[22] As pointed out by Bennett and Hendrix,[23] this clinical entity is poorly defined, with symptoms, x-ray changes, and manometric changes showing only variable and intermittent association.

PATHOGENESIS

As its name implies, the pathogenesis of SIDES is entirely unknown. A number of cases will show marked hypertrophy of the muscle layers of the esophagus, including longitudinal, circular, and muscularis mucosal layers.[24] The muscularis propria may reach a thickness of 2 cm. Auerbach's plexus may be infiltrated with chronic inflammatory cells.[25] However, the number of ganglion cells in this plexus is normal, in contrast to the decreased number seen in achalasia. Light microscopy reveals no abnormalities of the esophageal muscle.[26] One study has revealed wallerian degenerative changes in the peripheral branches of the vagus nerve.[26] The significance of these changes remains unclear.

Despite the normal number of ganglion cells in Auerbach's plexus, the hypersensitive response to extrinsic cholinergic stimulation in some patients with SIDES suggests that esophageal denervation may play a role in the genesis of this disorder.[22, 27] The isolated single case showing possible progression of SIDES to classic achalasia,[28] the description of "vigorous achalasia" as an early form of achalasia,[10] and the hypersensitivity of some patients with SIDES to cholinergic agents have raised the possibility that SIDES is, in fact, a prodromal stage or early form of classic achalasia. However, the current confusion about the pathogenesis of SIDES, the absence of the typical histopathological changes of achalasia, and the relatively normal LES function in these patients (described earlier) make this hypothesis unproven at the present time.

CLINICAL MANIFESTATIONS*

It is of paramount importance to obtain a detailed history in patients suspected of having SIDES, since it is the patient's complaints that should lead the clinician to the correct diagnosis. Correlative radiographic and manometric studies should be used to confirm the diagnosis made on the basis of the history alone. If one insists that the typical symptoms, radiographic abnormalities, and manometric

---

*See Table 8–5.

TABLE 8–5. *Clinical Manifestations of SIDES*

Esophageal colic
Occasional dysphagia
Occasional odynophagia
Nasal or oral regurgitation
Association of "triggering" stimuli
    Emotional stress
    Hot or cold liquid ingestion
    Gastroesophageal reflux

changes must all coexist to establish the diagnosis, then SIDES is an extremely rare entity.[7]

The typical patient with SIDES is a man or woman of any age, usually over 50, who may be a particularly anxious individual and who complains of symptoms during periods of emotional stress. The most typical symptom is esophageal colic occurring with swallows or during periods of rest and characterized by moderate to severe substernal chest pain radiating bilaterally to the anterior chest. The pain is similar to that of angina pectoris or myocardial infarction and may cause considerable clinical confusion in this regard.[7, 29] Useful distinguishing points in the patient with SIDES are absence of typical cardiac pain upon exertion, the occasional development of esophageal colic with swallowing, and the occasional occurrence of dysphagia and odynophagia. However, the distinction between cardiac and esophageal pain is a difficult one to make.[30]

Additional complaints in SIDES may include dysphagia, odynophagia, or regurgitation. These symptoms and the symptom of esophageal colic may be triggered by a variety of noxious environmental stimuli. These include emotional stress, ingestion of hot or cold liquids, and gastroesophageal reflux. The clinician should always attempt to define the factors that precipitate the patient's discomfort, since the first step in management is the removal of such factors.

The physical examination is unremarkable in patients with SIDES.

EVALUATION

Medical examination of the patient with SIDES should be tailored to the patient's initial complaint. For instance, most patients with this disorder will complain of chest pain. Routine chest x-ray and resting 12-lead electrocardiogram should be performed. Exercise electrocardiography and coronary arteriography may be required in certain individuals to exclude any possibility of arteriosclerotic heart disease.

Evaluation of the esophagus should include radiographic, endoscopic, and manometric studies. An esophagogram and upper gastro-

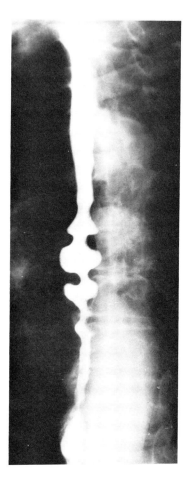

Figure 8-7.   Esophagogram in a patient with
SIDES. "Curling" of the barium column occurs
with the high pressure simultaneous contractions.

intestinal series (optimally done with cine studies) may reveal "curling" of the esophageal contour or segmentation of the barium column
(Fig. 8–7). In most instances, the peristaltic wave proceeds normally
down to the level of the aortic arch, where it breaks up into purposeless, segmented activity. These nonperistaltic (tertiary) contractions
are most prominent in the distal esophagus. In most cases, the esophagus is not dilated and empties normally once the barium reaches the
level of the LES. Occasionally, an epiphrenic diverticulum is observed.[29]

Since lesions infiltrating the esophageal wall or obstructing bolus
propagation may lead to the radiographic picture described above,
patients suspected of having SIDES should undergo endoscopy. The
area of the gastric fundus and LES should be carefully examined, and

TABLE 8–6. *Manometric Features of SIDES*

UES
    Normal findings
ESOPHAGEAL BODY
    Proximal striated muscle esophagus usually normal. However,
    entire esophagus may be involved.
    Most swallows followed by nonperistaltic (tertiary) waves
    in distal esophagus. Some normal peristalsis persists.
    Distal esophageal waves are of very high pressure, long
    duration, and multi-phasic contour.
    Spontaneous, nonperistaltic, high pressure waves occur
    without swallows.
LES
    Usually normal function.
    Occasional high resting pressure or incomplete relaxation.

biopsies should be performed on suspicious esophageal mucosal lesions.

Esophageal manometry is the logical final step in the diagnostic evaluation (Table 8–6). Typically, esophageal motility studies reveal normal UES function. The proximal striated muscle esophagus is also usually normal, showing peristaltic waves of normal contour and amplitude. However, the entire esophagus may be involved in the motor

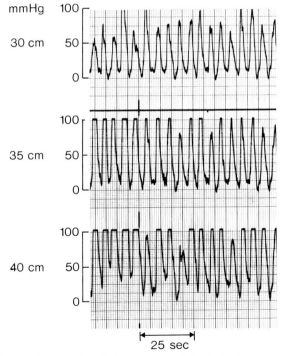

Figure 8-8. Motility study of the esophageal body in SIDES. High pressure simultaneous and spontaneous contractions are seen. The patient developed chest pain at the time this tracing was obtained.

TABLE 8–7.   Treatment of SIDES

Removal of "triggering" stimuli
    Emotional stress
    Hot, cold, carbonated beverage ingestion
    Gastroesophageal reflux
Use of short- or long-acting nitrites
Possibly pneumatic dilatation (not of proved efficacy)
Long (extended) esophagomyotomy in unresponsive patients with
incapacitating symptoms

---

disturbance. The smooth muscle esophagus frequently shows marked abnormalities of wave peristalsis, amplitude, and contour.[7, 22] While some normal peristalsis remains in the distal esophagus, most swallows are followed by nonpropagative (tertiary), high pressure, multiphasic waves. In addition, similar abnormal waves appear spontaneously without swallows (Fig. 8–8). These esophageal body abnormalities may not be observed if the patient is studied during an asymptomatic interval. Furthermore, some patients will not show these findings unless esophageal irritation occurs, as with the infusion of hydrochloric acid or other noxious agents.

Some patients will develop chest pain and the typical manometric features of SIDES during the procedure. This coupling of symptoms and manometric abnormalities establishes that the pain is of esophageal origin.[30] However, the instances in which chest pain has been associated with typical manometric changes of SIDES have been rare in our experience and in the experience of others. LES function is probably normal in most patients with SIDES,[31] but high LES resting pressure or incomplete LES relaxation has been described[7, 22] (Table 8–6).

As in achalasia, a few patients will demonstrate hypersensitivity to cholinergic agents. However, the presence of some normal distal esophageal peristalsis and a generally normally functioning LES make the diagnosis of achalasia untenable.

It should be emphasized that SIDES is a diagnosis made on the basis of the patient's history by careful delineation of the symptoms. Since radiographic and manometric abnormalities typical of SIDES may be seen in patients who do not have this syndrome, and since the x-ray and motility studies in patients with SIDES may be normal during asymptomatic intervals, these studies should be used only to help confirm the diagnosis and not to refute it.

TREATMENT*

Management of the patient with SIDES should always start with an attempt to remove stimuli that may be provoking symptoms. Partic-

---

*See Table 8–7.

ular attention should be paid to avoiding controversial topics or rapid eating during the dinner hour. Dealing with the patient's underlying chronic stress may help in certain instances. If hot, cold, or carbonated beverages trigger attacks, these should be avoided. Finally, some patients with symptoms of gastroesophageal reflux may develop additional symptoms of esophageal colic. It seems prudent to manage such patients initially with antacids and antireflux maneuvers.

Both short- and long-acting nitrites have been shown to be efficacious in selected patients with SIDES. Improvement in symptoms and correction of the manometric abnormality has been described with use of these agents[32, 33] (Fig. 8–9). Sublingual nitroglycerin may be used for isolated random attacks of pain that occur at infrequent intervals. Long-acting nitrites may be used in patients whose attacks are more frequent. In general, patients with SIDES have a more delayed response to nitrites than do patients with angina pectoris. Nitrite therapy is less effective in patients whose SIDES is triggered by gastroesophageal reflux.[33] Aggressive control of the reflux is the appropriate management in that case.

Vigorous pneumatic dilatation of the LES has been described in treatment of patients with SIDES. Usually more frequent dilatations are required with SIDES than with achalasia.[34] There are insufficient data to recommend this form of therapy. It is possible that successes occurred in patients who had coexistent LES dysfunction. Theoretically, one would not expect symptoms attributable to disordered esophageal peristalsis to disappear with brusque dilatation of the LES. Further studies of this mode of treatment are needed.

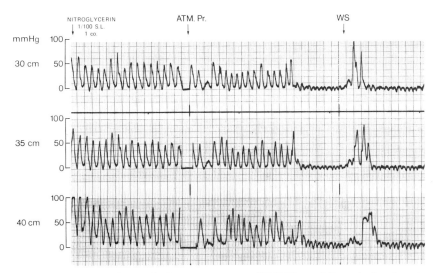

Figure 8-9. Motility study showing response of SIDES to sublingual nitroglycerin. Diminution in the spontaneous motor activity is seen. (*ATM. Pr*, momentary opening of system to atmospheric pressure; *WS*, wet swallow.)

When all else fails, and the patient's symptoms are incapacitating, or clearly adversely influencing his or her life style, a long esophagomyotomy should be considered.[35, 36] The particular type of surgery is partially dictated by the function of the LES. If the LES is normal, it should not be incised. If LESP is low, one needs to consider an antireflux procedure in addition to the myotomy. The myotomy itself usually involves the distal two-thirds of the esophagus up to the transverse aorta. If the motility disturbance extends into the skeletal muscle esophagus, then a total esophageal myotomy is required. The length of the incision is dictated by the location of the motor abnormality given by the preoperative esophageal motility study. While the results from the Mayo Clinic series are encouraging,[36] the rate of success in alleviating symptoms is not as great as with the modified Heller's myotomy performed for achalasia.

ESOPHAGEAL SCLERODERMA

PATHOGENESIS

While esophageal scleroderma is uncommon, it represents a model of esophageal dysfunction mediated by collagen disease and Raynaud's phenomenon (RP). The pathogenesis of the esophageal lesion in scleroderma is unknown, although several theories have been put forward to explain the observed motility disturbance. In pathologic studies of the lesion, atrophy of the smooth muscle and collagen deposition in the submucosa both occur to varying degrees in the distal two-thirds of the esophagus. The ganglionic plexuses are usually normal both in number and in histological appearance. The smaller arterial vessels may show intimal proliferation. Depending upon the degree of LES hypotension, varying degrees of gross and microscopic esophagitis may be present. Except in far-advanced cases, the proximal striated muscle esophagus is normal.[37, 38, 39]

The esophageal motor disturbance in scleroderma includes almost invariable loss of coordinated peristalsis in the distal two-thirds of the esophagus, decreased amplitude of the esophageal body waves, and reduction or absence of LES resting pressure. These three abnormalities may occur singly or together and may remain stable for years or show progression.[38, 40] Again, this disturbance almost always affects the distal two-thirds of the esophagus and spares the oropharynx, hypopharynx, UES, and cervical skeletal muscle esophagus. The motility dysfunction is poorly correlated with the pathologic findings and may antedate histologic abnormalities.[37]

Raynaud's phenomenon (RP) occurs in 80 to 90 percent of patients with scleroderma[41] and is the single most important clinical finding associated with the esophageal motor disturbance in this disease.[42] RP is closely correlated with the loss of esophageal peristalsis in scleroderma, and its presence strongly suggests esophageal involvement and possibly involvement of the less commonly affected sites in the gastrointestinal tract. Of note is the fact that when RP occurs as an isolated entity or with diseases other than scleroderma, loss of normal, coordinated esophageal body peristalsis is a common finding in most of the patients who have been studied.[42]

A recent study has shown that while RP closely correlates with loss of esophageal peristaltic activity, it does not correlate with esophageal function reflecting smooth muscle strength (wave pressure amplitude in the esophageal body or LES resting pressure).[43] The presence of, duration of, and severity of RP do not seem to influence the contractile strength of the smooth muscle esophagus. The implication of this study is that the motility disturbances in esophageal scleroderma may be mediated by two processes. The first process, associated with RP, results in loss of peristalsis. The close association of RP with the loss of esophageal peristalsis may be the result of several factors: ischemia of the vagus nerve, postganglionic neuronal ischemia, ischemia of smooth muscle with impairment of membrane conduction, and finally, the result of hyperadrenergic "overdrive" with impairment of normal vagally derived peristalsis. The second process, which may lead to the loss of smooth muscle contractile strength, is the smooth muscle atrophy and submucosal collagen deposition frequently seen in this disease. This process of atrophy and fibrosis may weaken the muscle itself or may diminish the responsiveness of the smooth muscle to intrinsic neural stimuli.

In studying patients with scleroderma and RP, Cohen and colleagues noted a diminished response of the LES to cholinesterase inhibitors and to gastrin I (agents that increase the concentration of acetylcholine at the smooth muscle membrane surface).[44] By contrast, the LES responded normally to a direct smooth muscle stimulant (methacholine). Cohen's study suggests that the esophageal smooth muscle weakness in scleroderma may be the result of resistance of the smooth muscle membrane to acetylcholine, rather than an inability of the muscle itself to contract. More work is needed to delineate the esophageal motor dysfunction of this complex disease.

CLINICAL MANIFESTATIONS

Most patients with scleroderma do not have esophageal symptoms until LES hypotension supervenes. Up to the time when the LES fails, the esophagus usually empties by gravity without difficulty. However, once the LES resting pressure is low, gastroesophageal reflux with its attendant symptoms and complications occurs (see Chapter 9). The degree of esophageal injury by acid and pepsin in

scleroderma is more severe than in the usual forms of gastroesophageal reflux. The degree of esophageal injury is increased due to the fact
that in addition to LES hypotension, secondary peristalsis is absent in
scleroderma. Therefore, the acid-clearing mechanism of the esophagus is impaired, and severe injury may result.[45]

Because of this impairment, patients with scleroderma who have
gastroesophageal reflux are very prone to develop severe heartburn,
bleeding esophagitis or esophageal ulcer, and severe peptic stricture
that may involve one-third to one-half of the esophagus. Heartburn,
dysphagia, odynophagia, pulmonary soilage, and weight loss may
occur in these patients. The weight loss may not only result from the
marked reduction in caloric intake secondary to dysphagia but may
also reflect coexistent malabsorption secondary to small bowel bacte-
rial overgrowth. Other gastrointestinal symptoms observed in these
patients include constipation or diarrhea and gastrointestinal bleeding, the last generally reflecting severe esophagitis.[46] Coexistent pulmonary, cardiac, renal, and rheumatologic involvement will influence
the clinical picture and the prognosis.

EVALUATION

Esophageal scleroderma is usually diagnosed when a patient
complains of heartburn, dysphagia, or weight loss. The most useful
initial study is an upper gastrointestinal series performed with or
without cine studies. This will usually demonstrate normal esophageal peristalsis down to the level of the aortic arch, at which point the
peristaltic wave is broken up into purposeless tertiary contractions.
The esophagus may be dilated and will be markedly distended if a
coexistent distal stricture is present. At times the esophagus and
stomach will appear as a common conduit because of the absence of
LES resting tone. Stricture formation, when present, is usually severe
and extends over a significant distance. Distal esophageal ulceration
may be present[47, 48] (Fig. 8–10).

Most patients with scleroderma and complaints of dysphagia
should undergo endoscopy to assess the severity of esophagitis and to
determine whether or not stricture formation is occurring. The esophageal mucosa will reveal varying degrees of esophagitis. The esophagitis is usually severe, demonstrating both friability and spontaneous bleeding. Deep esophageal ulceration may be present. A tough,
fibrous peptic stricture may be observed, precluding further passage
of the instrument. Such strictures are almost always benign, but histologic and cytologic evaluation should always be carried out to exclude cancer.[49]

Manometric evaluation of the esophagus in scleroderma is useful
to assess the stage of progression of the motor disturbance. This motor

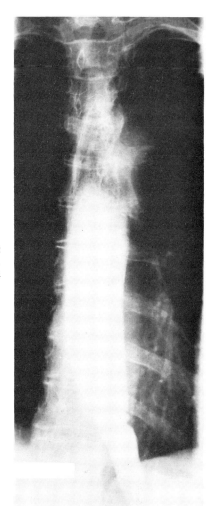

Figure 8-10. Esophagogram of patient with scleroderma. The esophagus is dilated. The gastroesophageal junction is patulous. A small distal esophageal ulcer is noted.

disturbance is highly variable in different patients and does not depend upon the duration of the disease nor upon the duration or severity of the Raynaud's phenomenon. Various patterns of esophageal motility emerge. In our experience, four patterns of motility disturbance have been observed[43] (Fig. 8–11 and Table 8–8).

First, an exceedingly rare type of patient with scleroderma and RP has normal esophageal body motility with normal peristalsis. This is extremely unusual because almost all patients with scleroderma and RP will have absence of normal esophageal peristalsis. In a second form of motility disorder, peristalsis is lost but wave amplitude and LES function are retained. In a third form, all esophageal body function is lost, but LES tone remains. Finally, in a fourth pattern, the smooth muscle esophagus is completely paralyzed, with loss of all

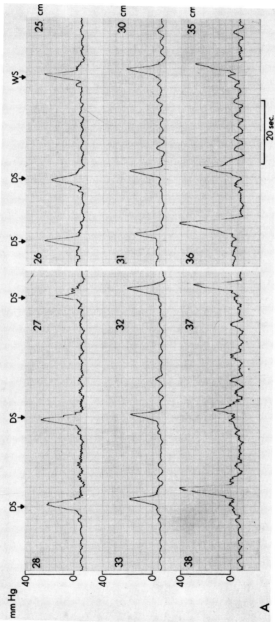

Figure 8-11. Patterns of esophageal motility in scleroderma. A, Normal motility in body of esophagus. LES function was essentially normal in this patient, except for a reduction in mean pressure (9.3 mm Hg). (DS, dry swallow.) B, Loss of coordinated peristalsis in esophageal body. Esophageal waves are of normal pressure, and the LES is normal (WS, wet swallow).

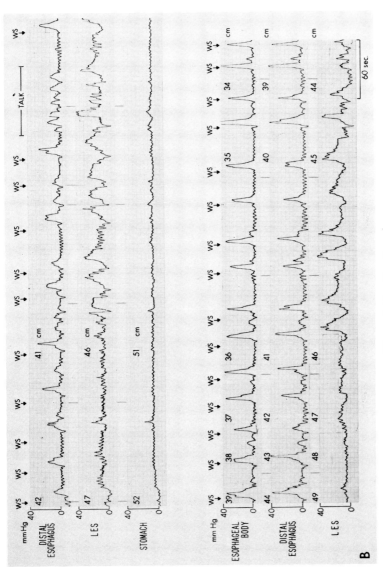

Figure 8-11. Continued.   Illustration continues on following page

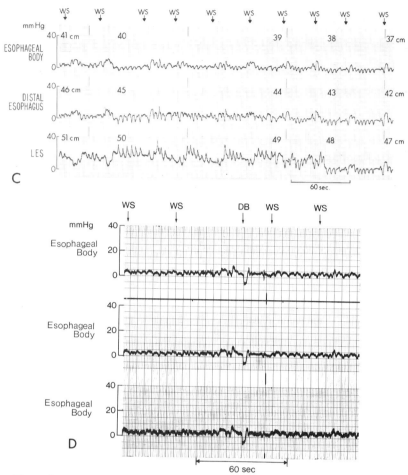

Figure 8-11. Continued. C, Loss of coordinated peristalsis and wave pressure in the esophageal body. The LES is normal. *D*, Total paralysis of smooth muscle esophagus. Coordinated peristalsis, esophageal wave pressure, and LES pressure are essentially absent (*DB*, deep breath). (Reprinted from Hurwitz A. L., Duranceau A., Postlethwait R. W.: Esophageal dysfunction and Raynaud's phenomenon in patients with scleroderma. Am. J. Dig. Dis., 21:601-606, 1976. By permission of Plenum Publishing Corporation, New York.)

TABLE 8–8. *Esophageal Motility Patterns in Scleroderma*

PATTERN	COORDINATED PERISTALSIS	NORMAL DISTAL ESOPHAGEAL WAVE PRESSURE	NORMAL LES PRESSURE
I (very rare)	+	+	−
II	−	+	+
III	−	−	+
IV	−	−	−

(Reprinted from Hurwitz A. L., Duranceau A., Postlethwait R. W.: Esophageal dysfunction and Raynaud's phenomenon in patients with scleroderma. Am. J. Dig. Dis., 21:601–606, 1976. By permission of Plenum Publishing Corporation, New York.)

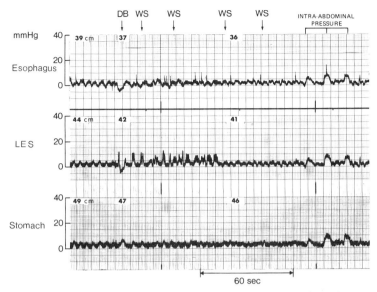

Figure 8-12. Slow pull-through motility study of gastroesophageal junction in scleroderma. No LES is identified. Increased intra-abdominal pressure is directly transmitted to the thoracic esophagus (*DB*, deep breath; *WS*, wet swallow.)

wave activity and complete absence of LES resting pressure. The clinician cannot determine a priori into which of these four patterns the patient falls. This is owing to the highly variable progression of the disease in different individuals. Measurements of pH performed in the distal esophagus may show a significant degree of acid reflux in the recumbent position. UES function is normal.

The esophageal motility study in scleroderma allows the clinician to assess the progression of the disease and can assist in the future management of the patient. In particular, absence of LES resting pressure in conjunction with absence of normal peristalsis is a warning that the complications of gastroesophageal reflux will take place (Fig. 8–12). When these manometric abnormalities are present, it is best to manage such patients with antacids and antireflux maneuvers, even if they are in an asymptomatic stage of the disease.

TREATMENT

There is no specific treatment for esophageal scleroderma.[7] Once LES hypotension occurs, and certainly once the patient develops esophageal symptoms, management with frequent antacids and with specific antireflux maneuvers should be carried out. The complications of gastroesophageal reflux, such as peptic stricture, should be managed conservatively, and only rarely should antireflux surgery be performed. Although some surgeons have advocated various forms of antireflux operations,[50] caution should be used since the absence of esophageal peristalsis may prevent emptying of the esophagus after such a procedure. Therefore, esophagitis and esophageal ulcer are best managed with antireflux maneuvers and antacids, and esophageal stricture is generally managed by bougienage.

The use of cholinergic agents, such as Urecholine, in patients with esophageal scleroderma has not been reported. Because these agents may increase LES resting pressure as well as enhance esophageal emptying, they may be efficacious in this disease.[51] However, once the LES has been structurally damaged, such drugs may be of no effect. Metoclopramide hydrochloride may also be efficacious in selected patients with esophageal scleroderma by increasing LES pressure and by enhancing the acid-clearing capability of the esophagus.[52] Trials with both of these classes of agents should be performed. The use of the new H_2 blocker, cimetidine, in the management of esophageal scleroderma may be highly effective through its well-known ability to reduce gastric acidity. Another method of controlling gastric acid production in esophageal scleroderma is by gastric irradiation, which may be very useful in this setting. The poorly documented effect of intra-arterial reserpine on improving coordinated esophageal peristalsis in esophageal scleroderma has not been pursued in terms of clinical efficacy.[53]

MISCELLANEOUS DISORDERS

While achalasia, SIDES, and esophageal scleroderma are the most significant prototypic diseases of deranged esophageal peristalsis, many other diseases produce disturbances in peristalsis. A classification of such disorders is possible according to their localization along the neuromuscular axis (Table 8–9).

CENTRAL NERVOUS SYSTEM DISEASE

Central nervous system disease may produce a reduction in the number of normal peristaltic waves following swallows or a reduction in esophageal wave pressure. These perturbations in esophageal peristalsis are probably caused by bilateral damage to the vagus nerve at the nuclear or supranuclear level. Vascular lesions of the central nervous system, including pseudobulbar palsy and other cerebrovascular accidents, may lead to a reduction in esophageal body peristalsis. In addition, degenerative diseases and demyelinating diseases, such as Parkinson's disease, amyotrophic sclerosis, and multiple sclerosis, may also produce marked reduction in peristalsis or absence of

TABLE 8–9. *Diseases Producing Disordered Peristalsis*

CENTRAL NERVOUS SYSTEM
      Vascular (cerebrovascular accident, pseudobulbar palsy)
      Degenerative (Parkinson's disease)
      Demyelinating (amyotrophic lateral sclerosis, multiple sclerosis)
      Miscellaneous (brainstem, cerebellar damage)
PERIPHERAL NEUROPATHY
      Diabetic
      Alcoholic
DISEASES OF THE INTRAMURAL ESOPHAGEAL GANGLIA
      Reduction in number of ganglia
            Idiopathic (achalasia)
            Toxic (Chagas' disease)
            Neoplastic destruction (e.g., retrograde extension of gastric cancer)
      "Irritation" of ganglia
            Gastroesophageal reflux
            Candidal esophagitis
            Caustic ingestion
            Psychological stress
DISEASES OF THE MOTOR END-PLATE
      Myasthenia gravis
MYOPATHIES
      Skeletal muscle (polymyositis, dermatomyositis)
      Smooth muscle (scleroderma, Raynaud's phenomenon, muscular dystrophies)
      Metabolic (e.g., thyrotoxicosis)

peristalsis in the esophageal body. Other lesions, especially those that result in brainstem or cerebellar damage, may also reduce orderly peristalsis following swallows.[54] On occasion, central nervous system disease may also produce dysfunction in both esophageal sphincters;[54, 55] these additional sphincteric abnormalities may then produce significant symptoms.

PERIPHERAL NEUROPATHY

Peripheral neuropathy of both the diabetic[56] and the alcoholic[57] have resulted in a reduction in normal esophageal body peristalsis. While other neuropathies may produce disordered peristalsis, they have not been well documented.

"Presbyesophagus" is a term originally coined by Soergel and colleagues to define esophageal peristaltic abnormalities noted in the elderly.[58] These workers found a reduction in the number of primary waves in patients 90 to 97 years of age when compared with controls. Additional defects of secondary peristalsis and LES function were also observed. A number of the elderly patients studied, however, had a variety of central nervous system or peripheral nerve diseases that could have influenced esophageal motility. A recent study of patients without neuromuscular disease has shown that elderly individuals have more peristaltic defects than younger persons. These defects include a greater number of "nonresponses" to swallows, more repetitive contractions, and more simultaneous contractions.[59] In contrast, another investigation of elderly men without neurologic disease showed no abnormalities of esophageal body peristalsis other than a reduction in absolute wave pressure amplitude.[60] Differences in patient selection and manometric criteria may explain some of the discrepancies in these various studies.

DISEASES OF THE INTRAMURAL ESOPHAGEAL GANGLIA

Achalasia and Chagas' disease are characterized by a reduction in the number of motor ganglia in the esophageal body and in the LES. The distinction between achalasia and SIDES has been discussed earlier in this chapter. A group of poorly defined syndromes sharing some of the features of achalasia defies precise classification. As previously mentioned, patients with "vigorous achalasia" have *high* pressure synchronous waves in the esophageal body.[10] Another group of patients have dilated esophagi but normal peristalsis and normal LES function on manometric study.[61] Still another group demonstrates hypertensive LES pressures and abnormal waves in the esophageal body but no esophageal dilatation.[62] Recent studies in patients with epiphrenic diverticula show several defects including incoordinate LES relaxation with the oncoming peristaltic wave, incomplete LES relaxation, and high pressure waves in the distal esophagus.[63] It is important not to be overly vigorous in classifying such "achalasia variants." Diagnosis and treatment should be guided by the specific findings of the esophageal motility study and not by a "label" attached to the motor disturbance.[7]

Marked disturbances of esophageal peristalsis may also occur when inflammatory or neoplastic disease of the esophagus damages the ganglia or local reflex arcs within the esophageal body wall. Gastroesophageal reflux may produce a variety of peristaltic abnormalities in the distal esophagus. These include an increase in tertiary contractions, an increase in spontaneous activity, an increase in resting tone in the esophageal body, and an increase in the duration of the esophageal contraction waves. These motor disturbances have been elegantly described by Siegel and Hendrix, who performed acid perfusion studies in patients with heartburn and in patients without heartburn.[64] On occasion, chest pain observed in patients with gastroesophageal reflux may be caused by these secondary motor abnormalities. Esophageal pseudodiverticula have appeared in conjunction with these motility disturbances and have been resolved when the underlying reflux esophagitis was effectively treated.[65] Candidal esophagitis and caustic ingestion may both produce a reduction in normal esophageal peristalsis, presumably because of a severe inflammatory change in the submucosa.[66, 67]

TABLE 8–10.   *Clinical Features of Invasive Malignancy Simulating Achalasia*

SIMILARITIES
    Esophageal dilatation
    Loss of propagative esophageal body peristalsis
    LES defects (hypertension, incomplete relaxation with swallows)
    Positive cholinergic response ("Mecholyl [methacholine chloride] test")
DISTINGUISHING FEATURES
    On occasion propagative peristalsis may be observed
    Endoscope usually cannot be passed through gastroesophageal junction
    Pathologic documentation of malignancy in biopsy or cytology specimens
    Occasional return of normal esophageal motor function after treatment[69]

Primary or contiguous carcinoma may produce peristaltic abnormalities owing to destruction of esophageal wall ganglia or nerve plexuses. Several cases of "esophageal achalasia" due to extension of adjacent carcinoma or sarcoma have been described.[68, 69, 70] Patients with malignancy invading the esophagus (usually retrograde spread of gastric cancer) may display many of the radiographic and manometric features of classic achalasia. These include esophageal dilatation, loss of peristalsis, LES abnormalities, and a positive cholinergic response. Important distinguishing points include the occasional presence of some orderly peristalsis, the inability of the endoscope to pass through the gastroesophageal junction, the pathologic demonstration of malignancy in biopsy or cytology specimens, and the occasional return to normal esophageal motor function after treatment.[69] The clinical features of invasive malignancy simulating achalasia are shown in Table 8–10.

DISEASES OF THE MOTOR END-PLATE

Myasthenia gravis, a disease of the skeletal muscle motor end-plate, may produce abnormal peristalsis, especially in the proximal skeletal esophagus. A reduction in wave amplitude in the proximal esophagus has also been described in patients with this disease. On occasion, a reduction in peristaltic wave frequency and wave amplitude is seen in the mid-esophagus in patients with myasthenia gravis.[54] The most disabling symptoms in this disease, however, result from the impairment of muscle function in the pharynx and UES (see Chapter 7).

MYOPATHIES

Myopathies may lead to deranged peristalsis in the esophagus. Idiopathic skeletal myopathies, such as polymyositis and dermatomyositis, usually produce deranged motor function at the level of the pharyngoesophageal junction and the UES.[55] Although not well-studied, anticipated additional findings include impairment of proximal skeletal muscle esophageal peristalsis, both in frequency of peristalsis and in amplitude of contractions. Idiopathic smooth muscle myopathic involvement occurs in scleroderma and in other collagen diseases associated with Raynaud's phenomenon. The muscular dystrophies may produce abnormal esophageal motility throughout the entire esophagus, since these diseases may affect both skeletal and smooth muscle. As an example, myotonic dystrophy may cause abnormalities of both UES function and of esophageal body peristalsis.[54, 71] Finally, thyrotoxic myopathy may also produce mixed skeletal and smooth muscle abnormalities. In thyrotoxicosis, both oropharyngeal dysphagia and deranged esophageal body peristalsis have been described.[54, 72]

CONCLUSION

Disorders of esophageal peristalsis may be caused by primary esophageal disease or by widespread systemic illness. These varied syndromes and diseases occur because of loss of central or peripheral control of esophageal peristaltic activity. Significant esophageal symptoms rarely occur unless high pressure simultaneous esophageal body contractions are present, or unless there is coexistent sphincter dysfunction. Clinical awareness of these disorders is crucial if the physician is to treat resultant complications, and if an adequate differential diagnosis of the dysphagias is to be developed.

REFERENCES

1. Diamant N. E., El-Sharkawy T. Y.: Neural control of esophageal peristalsis. A conceptual analysis. Gastroenterology, 72:546–556, 1977.
2. Earlam R. J., Ellis F. H., Nobrega F. T.: Achalasia of the esophagus in a small urban community. Mayo Clin. Proc., 44:478–483, 1969.
3. Earlam R. J.: Pathophysiology and clinical presentation of achalasia. Clin. Gastroenterol., 5(1):73–88, 1976.
4. Cassella R. R., Brown A. L., Sayre G. P., Ellis F. H.: Achalasia of the esophagus; Pathologic and etiologic considerations. Ann. Surg., 160:474–486, 1964.
5. Smith B.: The neurological lesion in achalasia of the cardia. Gut, 11:388–391, 1970.
6. Bettarello A., Pinotti H. W.: Oesophageal involvement in Chagas' disease. Clin. Gastroenterol., 5(1):103–117, 1976.
7. Pope C. E. 2nd: Motor disorders (of the esophagus). In: Gastrointestinal Disease. 2nd ed. (Sleisenger M. H., Fordtran J. S., eds.). W. B. Saunders Co., Philadelphia, 1978, pp. 513–537.
8. Cohen S., Lipshutz W., Hughes W.: Role of gastrin supersensitivity in the pathogenesis of lower esophageal sphincter hypertension in achalasia. J. Clin. Invest., 150:1241–1247, 1971.
9. Goyal R. K., Rattan S.: Nature of vagal inhibitory innervation to the lower esophageal sphincter. J. Clin. Invest., 55:1119–1126, 1975.

10. Sanderson D. R., Ellis F. H., Schlegel J. F., Olsen A. M.: Syndrome of vigorous achalasia. Clinical and physiologic observations. Dis. Chest, 52:508–517, 1967.
11. Ellis F. G.: The natural history of achalasia of the cardia. Proc. R. Soc. Med., 53:663–666, 1960.
12. Wychulis A. R., Woolam G. L., Anderson H. A., Ellis F. H.: Achalasia and carcinoma of the esophagus. J.A.M.A., 215:1638–1641, 1971.
13. Pierce W. S., MacVaugh H., Johnson J.: Carcinoma of the esophagus arising in patients with achalasia of the cardia. J. Thorac. Cardiovasc. Surg., 59:335–339, 1970.
14. Kraft A. R., Frank H. A., Glotzer D. J.: Achalasia of the esophagus complicated by varices and massive hemorrhage. N. Engl. J. Med., 288:405–406, 1973.
15. Mello M. H.: Return of esophageal peristalsis in idiopathic achalasia. Gastroenterology, 70:1148–1151, 1976.
16. Cannon W. B.: A law of denervation. Am. J. Med. Sci., 198:737–750, 1939.
17. Cohen S., Lipshutz W.: Lower esophageal dysfunction in achalasia. Gastroenterology, 61:814–820, 1971.
18. Bennett J. R., Hendrix T. R.: Treatment of achalasia with pneumatic dilatation. Mod. Treatment, 7:1217–1228, 1970.
19. Payne, S. W., Donoghue, F. E.: Surgical treatment of achalasia. Mod. Treatment, 7:1229–1240, 1970.
20. Jekler J., Lhotka J.: Modified Heller procedure to prevent postoperative reflux esophagitis in patients with achalasia. Am. J. Surg., 113:251–254, 1967.
21. Arvanitakis C.: Achalasia of the esophagus. A reappraisal of esophagomyotomy vs. forceful pneumatic dilation. Am. J. Dig. Dis., 20:841–846, 1975.
22. Kramer P.: Diffuse esophageal spasm. Mod. Treatment, 7:1151–1162, 1970.
23. Bennett J. R., Hendrix T. R.: Diffuse esophageal spasm. A disorder with more than one cause. Gastroenterology, 59:273–279, 1970.
24. Gillies M., Nicks R., Skyring A.: Clinical, manometric and pathological studies in diffuse oesophageal spasm. Br. Med. J., 2:527–530, 1967.
25. Nicks R., Gillies M., Skyring A.: Diffuse muscular spasm. (Diffuse muscular hypertrophy of the oesophagus.) Bull. Soc. Int. Chir., 6:637–648, 1968.
26. Cassella R. R., Ellis F. H., Brown A. L.: Diffuse spasm of the lower part of the esophagus. Fine structure of esophageal smooth muscle and nerve. J. A. M. A., 191:379–382, 1965.
27. Mellow M. M.: Symptomatic diffuse esophageal spasm. Manometric follow-up and response to cholinergic stimulation and cholinesterase inhibition. Gastroenterology, 73:237–240, 1977.
28. Kramer P., Harris L. D., Donaldson R. M.: Transition from symptomatic diffuse spasm to cardiospasm. Gut, 8:115–119, 1967.
29. Vantrappen G., Hellemans J.: Diffuse muscle spasm of the oesophagus and the hypertensive lower oesophageal sphincter. Clin. Gastroenterol., 5(1):59–72, 1976.
30. Brand D. L., Martin D., Pope C. E. 2nd: Esophageal manometrics in patients with angina-like chest pain. Am. J. Dig. Dis., 22:300–304, 1977.
31. DiMarino A. J., Cohen S.: Characteristics of lower esophageal sphincter function in symptomatic diffuse esophageal spasm. Gastroenterology, 66:1–6, 1974.
32. Orlando R. C., Bozymski E. M.: Clinical and manometric effects of nitroglycerin in diffuse esophageal spasm. N. Engl. J. Med., 289:23–25, 1973.
33. Swamy N.: Esophageal spasm: Clinical and manometric response to nitroglycerin and long-acting nitrites. Gastroenterology, 42:23–27, 1977.
34. Rider J. A., Moeller H. C., Puletti E. J., Desai D. C.: Diagnosis and treatment of diffuse esophageal spasm. Arch. Surg., 99:435–440, 1967.
35. Ellis F. H., Code C. F., Olsen A. M.: Long esophagomyotomy for diffuse spasm of the esophagus and hypertensive gastroesophageal sphincter. Surgery, 48:155–169, 1960.
36. Ellis, F. H., Olsen A. M., Schlegel J. F., Code C. F.: Surgical treatment of esophageal hypermotility disturbances. J. A. M. A., 188:862–866, 1964.
37. Treacy W. L., Baggenstoss A. H., Slocumb C. H.: Scleroderma of the esophagus. A correlation of histologic and physiologic findings. Ann. Intern. Med., 59:351–356, 1963.

38. Atkinson M., Summerling M. D.: Oesophageal changes in systemic sclerosis. Gut, 7:402–408, 1966.
39. Winship D. H.: Management of esophageal problems in patients with collagen vascular disorders. Mod. Treatment, 7:1241–1249, 1970.
40. Garrett J. M., Winklemann R. K., Schlegel J. F.: The course of esophageal deterioration in scleroderma. Mayo Clin. Proc., 46:92–96, 1971.
41. Winklemann R. K.: Classification and pathogenesis of scleroderma. Mayo Clin. Proc., 46:83–91, 1971.
42. Stevens M. B., Hookman P., Siegel C. I., Esterly J. R., Shulman L. E., Hendrix T.: Aperistalsis of the esophagus in patients with connective tissue disorders and Raynaud's phenomenon. N. Engl. J. Med., 270:1218–1222, 1964.
43. Hurwitz A. L., Duranceau A., Postlethwait R. W.: Esophageal dysfunction and Raynaud's phenomenon in patients with scleroderma. Am. J. Dig. Dis., 21:601–606, 1976.
44. Cohen S., Fisher R., Lipshutz W., Turner R., Myers A., Schumacher R.: The pathogenesis of esophageal dysfunction in scleroderma and Raynaud's disease. J. Clin. Invest., 51:2663–2668, 1972.
45. Atkinson M.: Oesophageal motor changes in systemic disease. Clin. Gastroenterol., 5(1):119–133, 1976.
46. Roseman D. M., Sleisenger M. H.: Systemic disease and the gut. *In: Gastrointestinal Disease.* 2nd ed. (Sleisenger M. H., Fordtran J. S., eds.). W. B. Saunders Co., Philadelphia, 1978, pp. 454–488.
47. Neschis M., Siegelman S. S., Rotstein J., Parker J. G.: The esophagus in progressive systemic sclerosis. A manometric and radiographic correlation. Am. J. Dig. Dis., 15:443–447, 1970.
48. Henderson R. D.: Scleroderma and related disorders. *In: Motor Disorders of the Esophagus.* (Henderson R. D., ed.). The Williams & Wilkins Co., Baltimore, 1976, pp. 170–176.
49. Matzner M. J., Trachtman B., Mandelbaum R. A.: Coexistent carcinoma and scleroderma of the esophagus. Am. J. Gastroenterol., 39:31–42, 1963.
50. Henderson R. D.: Treatment of scleroderma. *In: Motor Disorders of the Esophagus.* (Henderson R. D., ed.). The Williams & Wilkins Co., Baltimore, 1976, pp. 177–182.
51. Miller W. N., Ganeshappa K., Dodds W. J., Hogan W. J., Barreras R. F., Arndorfer R. C.: Effect of bethanechol on gastroesophageal reflux. Am. J. Dig. Dis., 22:230–234, 1977.
52. McCallum R. W., Ippolitti A. F., Cooney C., Sturdevant R. A. L.: A controlled trial of metoclopramide in symptomatic gastroesophageal reflux. N. Engl. J. Med., 296:354–357, 1977.
53. Willerson J. T., Thompson R. H., Hookman P., Herdt J., Decker J. L.: Reserpine in Raynaud's disease and phenomenon. Ann Int. Med., 72:17–27, 1970.
54. Fischer R. A., Ellison G. W., Thayer W. R., Spiro H. M., Glasser G. H.: Esophageal motility in neuromuscular disorders. Ann. Int. Med., 63:229–248, 1965.
55. Hurwitz A. L., Nelson J. A., Haddad J. K.: Oropharyngeal dysphagia. Manometric and cine esophagraphic findings. Am. J. Dig. Dis., 20:313–324, 1975.
56. Mandelstam P., Siegel C. I., Lieber A., Siegel M.: The swallowing disorder in patients with diabetic neuropathy-gastroenteropathy. Gastroenterology, 56:1–12, 1969.
57. Winship D. H., Caflisch C. R., Sboralski F. F., Hogan W. J.: Deterioration of esophageal peristalsis in patients with alcoholic neuropathy. Gastroenterology, 55:173–178, 1968.
58. Soergel K. H., Zboralski F. F., Amberg J. R.: Presbyesophagus: Esophageal motility in nonagenarians. J. Clin. Invest., 43:1472–1479, 1964.
59. Khan T. A., Shragge B. W., Crispin J. S., Lind E. J.: Esophageal motility in the elderly. Am. J. Dig. Dis., 22:1049–1054, 1977.
60. Hollis J. B., Castell D. O.: Esophageal function in elderly men. A new look at "presbyesophagus." Ann. Int. Med., 80:371–374, 1974.
61. Hogan W. J., Caflisch C. R., Winship D. H.: Unclassified oesophageal motor disorders stimulating achalasia. Gut, 10:234–240, 1969.
62. Code C. F., Schlegel J. F., Kelly M. L., Olsen A. M., Ellis F. H.: Hypertensive gastroesophageal sphincter. Mayo Clin. Proc., 35:391–399, 1960.

63. Meunier L., Duranceau A., Hurwitz A. L.: Lower esophageal sphincter (LES) dysfunction in patients with epiphrenic diverticula. Gastroenterology, 72:1101, 1977.
64. Siegel C. I., Hendrix T. R.: Esophageal motor abnormalities induced by acid perfusion in patients with heartburn. J. Clin. Invest., 42:686–695, 1963.
65. Bender M. K., Haddad J. K.: Disappearance of multiple esophageal diverticula following treatment of esophagitis. Gastrointest. Endosc., 20:19–22, 1973.
66. Lewicki A. M., Moore J. P.: Esophageal moniliasis: Review of common and less frequent characteristics. Am. J. Roentgenol. Radium Ther. Nucl. Med., 125:218–225, 1975.
67. Simeone J. F., Burrell M., Toffler R., Smith G. J. W.: Aperistalsis and esophagitis. Radiology, 123:9–14, 1977.
68. Kolodny M., Schrader Z. R., Rubin W., Hochman R., Sleisenger M. H.: Esophageal achalasia probably due to gastric carcinoma. Ann. Int. Med., 69:569–573, 1968.
69. Davis J. A., Kantrowitz P. A., Chandler H. L., Schatski S. C.: Reversible achalasia due to reticulum-cell sarcoma. N. Engl. J. Med., 293:130–132, 1975.
70. Herrera A. F., Colon J., Valdes-Dapena A., Roth J. L. A.: Achalasia or carcinoma? The significance of the mecholyl test. Am. J. Dig. Dis., 15:1073–1081, 1970.
71. Siegel C. I., Hendrix T. R., Harvey J. C.: The swallowing disorder in myotonia dystrophica. Gastroenterology, 50:541–550, 1966.
72. Leach W.: Generalized muscular weakness presenting as pharyngeal dysphagia. J. Laryngol. Otol., 75:237–240, 1962.

CHAPTER 9

DISORDERS OF THE LOWER ESOPHAGEAL SPHINCTER (LES)

INTRODUCTION

The normal lower esophageal sphincter (LES) is a zone of increased manometric pressure separating the esophagus from the stomach. Its function is to allow esophageal contents to pass into the stomach and to prevent the reflux of gastric and duodenal contents into the esophagus. As with all physiologic sphincters, distention proximal to the sphincter results in relaxation, whereas distention distal to it results in increased pressure in the sphincter. The normal LES has been discussed in Chapter 3. Figure 9–1 is a motility tracing from a normal LES.

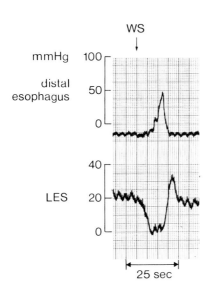

Figure 9-1. Normal lower esophageal sphincter. Resting pressure is 21 mm Hg. Relaxation to intragastric pressure is complete. The relaxation phase is well coordinated with the oncoming esophageal contraction. LES closes with a contraction that ends esophageal peristalsis. (*WS*, wet swallow.)

DETERMINANTS OF LESP

LES resting pressure (LESP) is not constant. Sphincter pressure varies from moment to moment in any one individual, and this variation in LESP may be marked. When one discusses "normal" values for LESP, one must take into consideration the many factors that affect this pressure. In recent years, literature on this subject has been voluminous. Information in this area is constantly changing, and only a brief description of some of the recent findings will be given. The poorly quantifiable effect of emotions on LESP has already been mentioned (Chapter 5).

Factors that may regulate LES function include neural, hormonal, myogenic, and mechanical influences, as well as certain drugs, foods, and other compounds.[1] Table 9–1 outlines these factors.

NEURAL.   Neural control is probably achieved through efferent fibers of both parasympathetic and sympathetic nerves. Inhibitory impulses carried in the trunk of the vagus nerve result in LES relaxation, and sympathetic impulses may antagonize this action.

HORMONAL.   Pharmacologic doses of hormones effect LESP. How physiologically important these hormonal effects may be is not yet clear. A thoughtful commentary on the present understanding of hormonal effects on LESP is found in Pope's recent review.[2]

MYOGENIC.   Intrinsic muscular activity in the LES has been demonstrated in opossum esophageal muscle strips. This intrinsic myogenic activity may be important in the regulation of LES resting muscle tone.

MECHANICAL.   Peri-hiatal structures such as the diaphragmatic crus, phrenoesophageal ligament, intra-abdominal esophageal segment, angle of His, and the mucosal rosette may affect LESP. The exact role of hiatal hernia in LES incompetence is controversial and will be discussed later in this chapter.

DRUGS, FOODS, AND OTHER FACTORS.   Additional environmental influences that affect LESP are discussed in detail below.

FACTORS CAUSING DECREASED LESP*

NEURAL.   There are conflicting data on the effect of vagotomy on LESP. Increased gastroesophageal reflux has been reported after vagotomy,[3] as well as decreased LES responsiveness to elevated intra-abdominal pressure.[4] A decrease in LESP following cervical vagotomy in dogs has been reported.[5] Both inhibitory and stimulatory effects of the cervical vagus on LESP have been demonstrated in the opossum, whereas no effect of the abdominal vagus on LES function was seen.[6]

---

*See Table 9–1.

TABLE 9–1. *Factors Regulating LESP*

FACTORS	INCREASED LESP	DECREASED LESP	UNCHANGED LESP
Neural	Cholinergic drugs Anticholinesterases Alpha-adrenergic agents	Intravenous atropine Beta-adrenergic agents Vagotomy (in animals) Alpha-adrenergic antagonists	Oral atropine Vagotomy (humans)
Hormonal	Gastrin Prostaglandin F_2A Motilin Bombesin	Secretin Cholecystokinin Glucagon Progesterone Estrogen Prostaglandin E_1, E_2, A_2	
Myogenic	Resting muscle tone	Possibly aging Possibly diabetes	
Mechanical	Surgical correction	Hiatal hernia Abnormal phrenoesophageal ligament insertion Absent intra-abdominal esophageal segment Nasogastric tube	
Drugs	Coffee Urecholine Methacholine hydrochloride Edrophonium Metoclopramide Betazole Metiamide	Theophylline Nicotine Alcohol Epinephrine Isoproterenol Phentolamine Nitroglycerine	Caffeine Cimetidine
Foods	Protein	Fats Chocolate	
Other Factors	Gastric alkalinization Gastric distention	Gastrectomy, smoking, hypoglycemia, hypothyroidism, amyloidosis, pernicious anemia, epidermolysis bullosa, gastric acidification	Gastric alkalinization

Studies in humans have shown no effect of vagotomy in reducing LESP.[4, 7, 8, 9] There is no convincing evidence at this time for an effect of vagotomy on LESP in humans. Intravenous atropine produces a slight decrease in LESP when either infused or uninfused catheters are used.[10, 11] Oral atropine, however, has no demonstrable effect on LESP.[12] Adrenergic agents such as epinephrine, isoproterenol, and phentolamine reduce LESP.[1]

HORMONAL.   Many hormones have been investigated to discover their relationship to LES function. The effects noted are usually pharmacologic and, as such, represent responses to unphysiologic doses of the hormones. Secretin, cholecystokinin, and glucagon in pharmacologic doses appear to decrease LESP, to antagonize the increase in LESP by gastrin, or to exert both of these effects.[1] Whether or not these hormones have an effect on LESP in physiologic doses is uncertain. Both progesterone and estrogen have been shown to cause a decrease in LESP,[13, 14] as have certain prostaglandins (E_1, E_2, A_1).[1]

MYOGENIC.   The effects of aging and diabetes on decreasing LESP have been reported and may be caused by myogenic influences.[15] However, more recent studies show no effect of diabetes on LESP.[16]

MECHANICAL.   Alteration of the normal anatomy of the cardioesophageal zone may result in a decrease in LESP. An abnormal phrenoesophageal ligament insertion, an absent intra-abdominal segment of the esophagus, or a hiatal hernia may reduce LESP. Nasogastric tube placement may promote reflux by mechanical means.

DRUGS.   Drugs that lower LESP include theophylline, alcohol, nicotine, and nitroglycerine.[1]

FOODS.   Fats[17] and chocolate[18] cause a decrease in LESP.

OTHER FACTORS.   Smoking,[19] hypoglycemia,[20] hypothyroidism, amyloidosis, epidermolysis bullosa, and gastric acidification[21] have all been reported to cause a decrease in LESP. One study showed that gastrectomy without vagotomy increased the incidence of gastroesophageal reflux,[22] but this observation has not been substantiated.

FACTORS CAUSING INCREASED LESP*

NEURAL.   Cholinergic agents such as Urecholine and methacholine raise LESP.[1] Edrophonium bromide, an anticholinesterase drug, and alpha-adrenergic agents have been shown to increase LESP.

HORMONAL.   The physiologic role of hormones in raising LESP remains controversial.[2] Exogenous gastrin increases LESP but only in unphysiologic (pharmacologic) doses.[23] It was initially thought that

---

*See Table 9–1.

gastric alkalinization caused increased gastrin levels that resulted in an increase in LESP. However, LESP and serum gastrin levels do not correlate well in patients who have high, low, or normal LESP values. Gastric alkalinization has not been shown to increase serum gastrin.[24] Feeding, however, appears to increase both LESP and gastrin, more so in normal controls than in those with gastroesophageal reflux.[25]

It would appear that high doses of exogenous gastrin do increase LESP, but at the present time there does not appear to be convincing evidence of any physiologic influence of gastrin on LESP. The difficulties in arriving at these conclusions are many, as described by Dodds et al.[26] Serum gastrin levels may not correlate well with those found in body tissue. Radioimmunoassay determinations may not measure biologically active gastrin and may not discriminate between the different molecular species of gastrin that are present. Lastly, gastrin may have an inotropic effect on LES contractility that is not linearly related to its serum concentration. In order to know what effect gastrin has on LESP, one may also need to know serum or tissue levels of inhibitory hormones such as secretin, cholecystokinin, and glucagon. The relationship of gastrin levels to LESP is made more confusing by the findings in patients with the Zollinger-Ellison syndrome (ZES) and with pernicious anemia. Elevated levels of serum gastrin are present in both conditions, but some ZES patients have increased LESP,[27] whereas patients with pernicious anemia have decreased LESP.[28]

Prostaglandin F_2A, motilin, and bombesin are other hormones shown to cause an elevation of LESP when given in pharmacologic doses.

MYOGENIC. The sphincter muscle appears to have intrinsic tone, and it behaves differently from adjacent circular muscle in the esophagus and stomach. Intrinsic myogenic factors appear to be important in the regulation of LES resting tone.

MECHANICAL. Surgical correction of anatomic defects may improve LESP by mechanical means. Such maneuvers include correcting abnormal phrenoesophageal ligament insertion, producing an intra-abdominal segment of esophagus, and fundoplication.

DRUGS. Coffee raises LESP, although caffeine has not been shown to have any effect on LESP.[29] Urecholine, methacholine, edrophonium bromide, metoclopramide hydrochloride, betazole, and metiamide, a histamine-2 blocker, have all been shown to cause an increase in LESP.[1]

FOODS. Protein meals increase LESP.[17]

OTHER FACTORS. Gastric alkalinization has been shown to increase LESP,[22] but some conflicting data on this point have been presented.[24] Gastric distention by itself has also been shown to increase LESP.

FACTORS SHOWN NOT TO ALTER LESP*

Recent studies using infused catheters show no effect of vagotomy on LESP in the human.[4, 7, 8, 9] Oral atropine[12] and caffeine[29] also do not affect LESP. Cimetidine, a new histamine-2-blocking drug, has not been shown to have any effect on LESP, in contrast to the LESP-increasing effect of metiamide.

CLINICAL DISORDERS OF LES FUNCTION

Disorders of LES function can be divided into two groups: those associated with a low LESP and attendant gastroesophageal reflux and those associated with high pressure and a poor or incoordinately relaxing lower esophageal sphincter. A low pressure LES does not present a barrier to gastroduodenal contents and permits reflux into the esophagus. Conversely, a hypertensive and incompletely or incoordinately relaxing sphincter poses a barrier to esophageal bolus propagation and prevents or delays food passage into the stomach, with resultant dysphagia.

GASTROESOPHAGEAL REFLUX

Gastroesophageal reflux remains one of the most important problem areas in which manometric studies are performed. The evaluation of patients with this disorder should include a careful understanding of the patient's symptomatology as related in his history. The history is usually sufficient to suggest that the patient truly has gastroesophageal reflux. There are, however, instances in which symptomatology is confusing and not entirely diagnostic. In such cases further studies are necessary to evaluate the patient's disease.

PATHOGENESIS

The situations in which gastroesophageal reflux occurs in conjunction with an incompetent LES are listed in Table 9–2. Low LESP is a common finding in all these disorders, although other factors may also be operative.

INFANCY. Vomiting and regurgitation due to gastroesophageal reflux are common problems in infants and young children. The syndrome of "chalasia" (relaxation of the LES) was postulated in 1947 to explain these findings.[30] Studies using uninfused catheters have

---

*See Table 9–1.

TABLE 9–2. *Causes and Clinicai Manifestations of Gastroesophageal Reflux*

CAUSES OF GASTROESOPHAGEAL REFLUX
  Infancy (chalasia)
  Pregnancy
  Oral contraceptives
  Ascites
  Esophagitis
  Scleroderma
  Pernicious anemia
  Idiopathic adult chalasia
  Hiatal hernia

CLINICAL MANIFESTATIONS OF GASTROESOPHAGEAL REFLUX
  Heartburn
  Regurgitation
  Waterbrash
  Halitosis
  Dysphagia
  Angina-like chest pain
  Pulmonary symptoms
  Anemia due to chronic blood loss
  Acute gastrointestinal bleeding
  Food impaction

shown that LESP is low in the first 6 months of life,[31] but more recent studies utilizing infused catheters suggest that normal infants have a well-developed LES by 2 weeks of age.[32] In these studies not all infants and children with gastroesophageal reflux had a low LESP. It is postulated that low LESP is not the sole determinant of gastroesophageal reflux in children. Infants and children with gastroesophageal reflux, however, usually have lower LESP than normal children of the same age. The presence of a hiatal hernia is not always correlated with the presence of gastroesophageal reflux in children.

PREGNANCY. Heartburn is a common symptom during pregnancy and is associated with a diminished LESP.[33] Pregnant women with heartburn have a lower LESP than pregnant women without heartburn.[34] LESP in these pregnant women returns to normal in the postpartum period. This decrease in LESP may be due to increased levels of progesterone, estrogen, or both during pregnancy.[35] Decreased LESP has likewise been demonstrated in women taking sequential oral contraceptives.

ASCITES. The role of ascites in promoting gastroesophageal reflux remains controversial. Earlier studies with uninfused catheters showed that patients with tense ascites often had low LESP and gastroesophageal reflux.[36] Recent studies using uninfused catheters have failed to show either any decrease in LESP in patients with ascites or any increase in this LESP after diuresis.[37]

ESOPHAGITIS. Esophagitis experimentally induced in cats results in a decrease in LESP, with return to normal values following healing of the esophageal inflammation.[38] Although it is usually reasoned that esophagitis is a result of low LESP and gastroesophageal reflux, these studies suggest that the reverse may also be true. Thus, LES hypotension with gastroesophageal reflux may result in esophagitis that in turn may result in a further decreased LESP, initiating a vicious cycle. Whether these studies in cats are applicable to humans remains to be demonstrated. Isolated cases exist in which LESP improves after treatment of esophagitis with antireflux measures.

SCLERODERMA.   Esophageal scleroderma is a smooth muscle disorder that affects function of the esophageal body and the LES. This disease is fully discussed in Chapter 8. LESP is frequently decreased in esophageal scleroderma, resulting in free reflux with severe esophagitis. The motor disorder of the smooth muscle portion of the esophageal body is associated with poor acid-clearing from the esophagus and further promotes the development of esophagitis. Stricture formation may also occur.

PERNICIOUS ANEMIA.   Patients with pernicious anemia have significantly lower LESP than normal subjects.[28] The sphincter response to intravenous pentagastrin is also reduced. Heartburn is not a common symptom in these patients, however, possibly because of associated achlorhydria. Esophagitis in such patients is usually due to bile reflux.[39]

IDIOPATHIC ADULT CHALASIA.   Probably the largest number of patients who demonstrate gastroesophageal reflux fall in this group. LES hypotension of unknown cause has been given the label of "idiopathic adult chalasia." The cause for the LES hypotension remains obscure. Whether decreased endogenous gastrin levels can be implicated in this LES hypotension remains an unsettled issue. Until more is known about the interrelation of the various hormones regulating sphincter pressure, this question will remain unresolved. Both intrinsic muscle abnormalities and extrinsic mechanical factors may produce reflux in these patients.

HIATAL HERNIA.   Hiatal hernia has long been implicated as a cause of gastroesophageal reflux. Reflux can occur in the absence of a hiatal hernia, and many patients with hiatal hernia do not have gastroesophageal reflux. The mere presence of a hiatal hernia detected in radiographic studies should not be taken as evidence for the presence of gastroesophageal reflux. Recent literature tends to minimize the role of hiatal hernia in causing gastroesophageal reflux.[40] Earlier studies using uninfused catheters have established manometric criteria for the diagnosis of hiatal hernia.[41] These criteria include: (1) increased LES length, (2) a plateau, at times with a proximal or distal peak, (3) double respiratory reversal, and (4) variability in configuration and length of the LES on repeated pull-throughs. The importance of diagnosing a hiatal hernia by manometric study seems less important than it did 10 years ago. LESP and the presence or absence of reflux appear to be more important data to obtain than whether or not a hiatal hernia is present.

CLINICAL MANIFESTATIONS*

By far the most common clinical manifestation of gastroesophageal reflux is heartburn. The severity of this symptom may not always be well correlated with the degree of esophagitis present. Heartburn may be intense when esophageal inflammation is minimal, and patients with long-standing, severe esophagitis may not have heartburn at all. Severely damaged mucosa may have diminished pain sensitivity through local nerve damage. Mucosal sensitivity to refluxed material must vary as does the appreciation of pain secondary to mucosal inflammation.

Heartburn may be intermittent, often occurring after a meal and induced by alcohol, hot coffee, citrus juices, or spicy foods. Some patients may note heartburn only when they lie flat in bed and some only when they lie on their left side. Regurgitation of acid contents into the mouth may be noted, especially with bending over, during straining maneuvers, or while lying flat in bed. Patients may also complain of a metallic, bitter, or salty taste in their mouths (waterbrash), and they may even complain of halitosis.

Dysphagia may be the presenting symptom of a patient with esophagitis. The food bolus may be felt to "stick" after swallowing. Often the patient can localize exactly the area where the bolus sticks, and this may give a clue as to the location of the abnormality. Dysphagia may be caused by mechanical obstruction to passage of the food bolus, such as occurs with an esophageal stricture, ring, or malignancy. Dysphagia, however, may occur in the absence of mechanical obstruction and may be seen in patients with esophagitis without stricture. In such cases dysphagia may be due to disordered motor activity in the esophagus or to mucosal inflammation. Absent or weak peristaltic activity as well as forceful nonpropulsive motor activity may be observed in patients with esophagitis.[42, 43] These motor disturbances may explain dysphagia in those cases in which stricture is not present.

The location of the obstruction is usually at or distal to the level where the patient feels the food "sticking." The area of obstruction is never proximal to the area localized by the patient. Thus, if the patient suggests that food sticks at the lower end of the sternum, the esophageal abnormality is usually located in the distal esophagus. If the patient feels that food sticks high in the chest, the abnormality may be

---

*See Table 9–2.

found at that level or anywhere distal to it. An interesting variant occurs in those patients who complain of food sticking in the throat or cervical esophagus and who may be suspected of having oropharyngeal dysphagia. A significant number of patients with gastroesophageal reflux may never complain of heartburn or regurgitation but simply of food sticking at the level of the cervical esophagus.[44] These patients do not have oropharyngeal dysphagia but do have an incompetent LES with reflux. The UES is found to function normally.[45] Symptoms seem to improve following antireflux treatment.

Odynophagia (painful swallowing) is a symptom that almost always signifies esophageal pathology and must be investigated fully. Globus hystericus, on the other hand, is not usually associated with esophageal pathology, and is felt to be a functional symptom. It is not dysphagia in the true sense of the word. It refers to the sensation of a "lump" in the throat constantly present and not affected by swallowing. One must be careful in making a diagnosis of globus, since the sensation of a lump in the neck or esophagus that occurs after a swallow and lasts for a long period of time suggests esophageal pathology and not globus. True dysphagia must never be labeled a functional symptom and must be carefully evaluated since it almost always signifies the presence of esophageal disease.

Chest pain simulating angina pectoris may occur in patients with esophagitis.[46] Associated symptoms, such as heartburn or regurgitation, may suggest that the cause of the chest pain is esophagitis rather than heart disease. Acid perfusion studies and treadmill exercise testing may be required to arrive at the true cause of the chest pain in such patients.

Nocturnal regurgitation may result in choking, coughing, or wheezing and may eventuate in chronic lung disease[47] (see Chapter 6).

Chronic blood loss and iron deficiency anemia as well as acute upper gastrointestinal bleeding may be the first presenting symptoms of esophagitis. Many such patients have never had symptoms of heartburn or regurgitation. If such symptoms did occur, they may have been ignored.

Impacted food in the esophagus with total esophageal obstruction may occasionally be the presenting symptom in patients with esophagitis. Very often such patients have had regurgitation or heartburn but have not paid attention to these symptoms. They may have had a mild sensation of food "sticking," but did not seek medical attention until progressive luminal narrowing produced distal esophageal food impaction. Usually such patients have developed fibrous strictures, although distal esophageal narrowing may be seen without true stricture formation in patients with severe esophagitis. Inflammation and edema of tissues may narrow the lumen sufficiently to cause obstruction to the food bolus.

EVALUATION OF GASTROESOPHAGEAL REFLUX

When the history is not diagnostic, various combinations of special studies may be necessary to evaluate patients with gastroesophageal reflux. In some instances a single test may be adequate, while in others many different studies may be required. Evaluation of patients suspected of having gastroesophageal reflux may include manometry, pH testing, acid perfusion studies, endoscopy and endoscopic biopsy, radiographic studies, and possibly recently introduced isotopic methods.

MANOMETRIC EVALUATION OF LESP. Although there is some evidence to the contrary,[48] the majority of investigators seem to agree that reflux is associated with a low LESP. The presence of reflux, as demonstrated by an intraesophageal pH electrode, is usually associated with low LESP.[49] High LESP values are usually not associated with reflux, whereas very low LESP's in the range of 0 to 10 mm Hg above gastric base line pressure usually are associated with reflux. Manometric studies that demonstrate an absent or very low LESP in a patient would certainly be consistent with the presence of gastroesophageal reflux (Fig. 9–2).

pH STUDIES. Measurement of sphincter pressure alone is insufficient to determine whether or not reflux is present. Overlap in LESP values occurs between normal individuals and those with gastroesophageal reflux. The use of an intraesophageal pH electrode gives

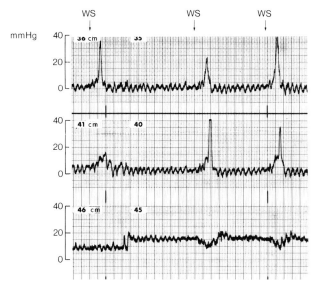

Figure 9-2. Hypotensive LES. The distal recording shows a resting LES pressure gradient of 5 mm Hg as the catheter is pulled from the stomach into the LES. The patient presented with symptoms of gastroesophageal reflux. (WS, wet swallow.)

more direct evidence of the presence or absence of reflux (see Chapter 5). pH studies may be done either at the time of manometric studies or as a separate procedure. Figures 5–2 through 5–5 in Chapter 5 illustrate findings in normal patients, in those with free reflux, and in those with reflux brought on by straining maneuvers. A positive test in which pH does not rise as the electrode is brought above the LES is consistent with the presence of gastroesophageal reflux. Many normal patients will intermittently demonstrate some gastroesophageal reflux, particularly during daytime hours, and especially in a postcibal state. Nocturnal reflux, however, is unusual in normal patients but is a common finding in those with clinically significant gastroesophageal reflux.[50] For this reason continuous pH monitoring (particularly nocturnal pH monitoring) has been suggested as a more effective method to determine whether or not significant gastroesophageal reflux is present.[51, 52]

ACID PERFUSION STUDIES. Acid perfusion studies (Bernstein test) may be performed in conjunction with manometric studies and have been discussed in Chapter 5. Esophageal motor dysfunction can be demonstrated manometrically during a positive acid perfusion test (Fig. 5–6, Chapter 5) and may be helpful in the evaluation of positive responses. A positive acid perfusion study indicates that the patient's symptoms are probably due to esophageal sensitivity to acid (possibly because of gastroesophageal reflux with resultant esophagitis). It has been suggested that patients with peptic disease may mimic a positive Bernstein test owing to gastric sensitivity to acid perfusion (Palmer test). There may be some instances in which confusion can arise through misinterpretation of such results.

ENDOSCOPY AND ENDOSCOPIC BIOPSY. Moderate and severe degrees of esophagitis are readily discernible at the time of endoscopy. The presence of mild esophagitis, however, may be difficult to determine visually at the time of endoscopy. Biopsy findings are not always well correlated with visual impression. In addition, esophagitis may be patchy in distribution, and the biopsy specimen itself may not truly reflect the actual pathologic state. Suction biopsy specimens may be more helpful than endoscopic biopsy specimens.[53] These factors must be taken into consideration in determining the role of endoscopy and biopsy in the evaluation of patients with reflux esophagitis. Histologic findings in moderate to severe esophagitis include epithelial ulceration and polymorphonuclear leukocytes in the lamina propria. Criteria for the diagnosis of mild to moderate esophagitis have been described as thickening of the basal epithelial layer and elongation of papillae.[54] These criteria are not, however, universally accepted.[55]

RADIOLOGY. Fluoroscopic evaluation of the esophagus utilizing liquid barium is helpful in ascertaining whether there are any structural lesions present such as stricture or malignancy. In addition, fluoroscopy may be useful to assess esophageal motor function. Gastroesophageal reflux is poorly demonstrated by such studies. Only a fairly marked degree of reflux is demonstrated by this method. Compared to intraesophageal pH studies, radiography is a relatively insensitive way of demonstrating gastroesophageal reflux. The use of acid barium was proposed as a method to separate those patients with esophagitis from normal patients, but this has not been found to be useful and has been largely abandoned.[56]

The presence of a hiatal hernia is best demonstrated by radiography. Whether or not hiatal hernia is causal in gastroesophageal reflux remains controversial, however.

GASTROESOPHAGEAL SCINTISCANNING.   Fisher et al. recently described gastroesophageal scintiscanning in normal individuals and in patients with gastroesophageal reflux.[57] This radioisotopic method proved to be a relatively noninvasive and reliable method to quantitate gastroesophageal reflux. Its use and clinical value in reflux evaluation remain to be determined.

ACID-CLEARING TEST.   Booth et al. proposed that patients with esophagitis do not clear the esophagus of acid as rapidly as do normal patients.[58] These impressions have been subsequently substantiated.[59] Altered peristalsis in the diseased esophagus or recurrent reflux of instilled hydrochloric acid may explain this impairment of esophageal clearing. This test is not at present very popular, and it is not certain how well it discriminates normal patients from those with esophagitis.

COMMON CAVITY TEST.   Some patients with gastroesophageal reflux may have negative pH and manometric studies. Butterfield et al. described the common cavity test as a further method to investigate the presence of reflux.[60] Increase in intraesophageal pressure as a response to abdominal compression was significantly greater in patients with gastroesophageal reflux compared with normal subjects. Addition of this study to the measurement of LESP and to pH determinations may be useful in studying patients with gastroesophageal reflux.

TREATMENT OF GASTROESOPHAGEAL REFLUX*

MEDICAL.   Relief of heartburn and healing of esophagitis may be accomplished by (1) combating reflux, (2) increasing sphincter competence, (3) reducing intraluminal acid content, or (4) increasing esophageal acid-clearing.

_____

*See Table 9–3.

TABLE 9–3.   *Treatment of Gastroesophageal Reflux*

MEDICAL
1. *Combat reflux*
   Elevate head of bed
   Reduce fluid intake after evening meal

2. *Increase sphincter competence*
   Avoid fats, chocolate, and caffeine in diet.
   Avoid tobacco and alcohol
   Avoid anticholinergic drugs
   Decrease intra-abdominal pressure
      Lose weight
      Avoid tight clothing, braces
      Avoid straining maneuvers
   Use drugs: Urecholine, metoclopramide

3. *Reduce intraluminal acid content*
   Use antacids
   Use histamine-2 antagonists (cimetidine)
   Radiate parietal mass

4. *Increase esophageal acid-clearing*
   Urecholine
   Metaclopramide

SURGICAL (SEE CHAPTER 10.)

(1) Combating Reflux.   Nocturnal reflux is a major problem in patients with gastroesophageal reflux, since reflux is usually maximal in the supine position. Antireflux treatment is achieved by elevation of the head of the bed on 6 inch blocks. This maneuver allows gravity to deter reflux and is probably the one most effective form of medical treatment. Unfortunately, it is often overlooked because of its minor inconvenience. Clinical data support the tenet that all other forms of medical therapy are generally much less effective when not used in conjunction with elevation of the head of the bed. Most patients can learn to sleep comfortably in this position and often note very prompt symptomatic improvement. Simply using large pillows or a bolster or wedge under the mattress ("cracking" the bed) is much less effective, and may actually make matters worse.

(2) Increasing Sphincter Competence.   Certain dietary measures, such as avoiding fats, chocolate, and caffeine, may increase LESP. Similarly, the avoidance of tobacco and alcohol may be beneficial. There is some evidence to suggest that anticholinergic drugs should not be used in patients with gastroesophageal reflux.[61]

Obesity, ascites, and pregnancy may cause gastroesophageal reflux because of increased intra-abdominal pressure, but recent studies cast some doubt on this mechanism. Thus, decreasing intra-abdominal pressure is an unproven method to improve sphincter competence. Weight loss seems to improve gastroesophageal reflux but by mechanisms that are not clear. Avoidance of tight girdles, back braces, and other such devices may diminish gastroesophageal reflux. Straining, such as with heavy lifting, results in a Valsalva maneuver and should be discouraged.

Cholinergic drugs such as Urecholine have been shown to increase LESP,[62] to ameliorate the symptoms of gastroesophageal reflux,[63] and to reduce acid-clearing time.[64] Undesirable side effects of these drugs include increased gastric acid production in some patients as well as sweating, salivation, and increased gastrointestinal motility. Metoclopramide hydrochloride, a drug that stimulates smooth muscle contraction, has also been demonstrated to increase LESP, but controlled studies on its effectiveness in treating patients with esophagitis are lacking.[65] Although metiamide, an early histamine-2 antagonist, was noted to increase LESP, recent studies with cimetidine demonstrate no effect on LESP.[66] Cimetidine, however, does improve the symptoms of gastroesophageal reflux.[67]

(3) Reducing Intraluminal Acid Content. Antacid therapy is another cornerstone of antireflux treatment. Antacids are probably effective in controlling symptoms and possibly effective in bringing about healing of esophagitis. Effectiveness of antacid therapy is potentiated by elevation of the head of the bed at night. Antacids seem to exert their effect by neutralizing gastric acid and possibly by increasing LESP through gastric alkalinization.[21] Dosage of antacids must be titrated and will vary depending upon the antacid used and the secretory state of the patient.

Histamine-2 receptor antagonists are potent inhibitors of gastric secretion and have recently been shown to be as effective as antacids in the treatment of duodenal ulcer. Their usefulness in the treatment of reflux esophagitis remains to be demonstrated.[67]

Radiation of the parietal mass is an effective method to reduce gastric secretion and may be beneficial in selected patients.

(4) Increasing Esophageal Acid-Clearing. In addition to their effect on improving sphincter competence, certain pharmacologic agents, such as Urecholine[64] and metoclopramide hydrochloride[65] have been shown to increase acid-clearing from the esophagus. Thus, these agents appear to have a dual role in the treatment of gastroesophageal reflux. It is also possible that healing of esophagitis in itself may result in improved peristaltic activity in the esophagus and lead to increased acid-clearing.

SURGICAL. Surgical treatment is usually reserved for those patients with severe reflux esophagitis not responsive to the usual forms of medical management. The indications for surgical treatment as well as the types of operations used will be discussed in detail in Chapter 10. The indications for surgery include severe symptoms refractory to medical therapy, stricture, bleeding, and recurrent pulmonary complications secondary to aspiration.

THE HYPERTENSIVE LES

A variety of clinical disorders may be associated with an LES that is hypertensive and partially relaxing or nonrelaxing or that relaxes in an incoordinate fashion with oncoming esophageal peristalsis. Patients who have a hypertensive LES that relaxes completely with swallows and that does so in a coordinate fashion with the oncoming peristaltic wave probably never have symptoms; therefore, isolated sphincter hypertension is of no clinical significance. Certainly patients with Zollinger-Ellison syndrome, who have normally relaxing hypertensive sphincters, do not have dysphagia. A full description of this syndrome has been presented in Chapter 8. Only a general overview of the LES dysfunction in these entities will be given here. Figure 9–3 demonstrates a hypertensive LES with only partial relaxation to gastric base line pressure following a swallow.

PATHOGENESIS*

ACHALASIA.   As stated in Chapter 8, achalasia is a disorder in which there is deranged motor activity in both the body of the esophagus and in the LES. Resting LESP in achalasia is usually considerably higher than normal and often is in the range of 40 to 80 mm Hg above gastric base line. Relaxation of this sphincter is incomplete following a swallow, so that a gradient always exists between the sphincter and gastric base line pressure (Fig. 9–4). A normal postdeglutitive contraction occurs in the sphincter. A reduction in LESP may be seen in patients with achalasia who have undergone pneumatic dilatation or esophagomyotomy.

GASTROESOPHAGEAL REFLUX WITH OR WITHOUT HIATAL HERNIA.   A hypertensive or hypercontracting sphincter may be seen, usually transiently, in patients with gastroesophageal reflux (Fig. 9–5).

---

*See Table 9–4.

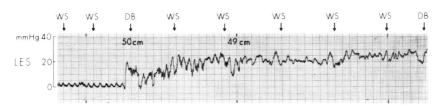

Figure 9-3.   Lower esophageal sphincter in a patient with achalasia. When the motility tube is pulled from the stomach into the sphincter, the resting pressure there is at the upper limits of normal (25 mm Hg above gastric pressure). Incomplete or absent relaxation is observed with swallows. (WS, wet swallow; DB, deep breath.)

TABLE 9–4. *Causes of the Hypertensive LES*

Achalasia
Gastroesophageal reflux with or without hiatal hernia
Association with diffuse esophageal spasm
Idiopathic LES dysfunction (hypertensive, hypercontracting, nonrelaxing)
Association with diverticula (? cause or effect)

Transient sphincter hypertension may occur as a sequela of acid reflux. Because of this phenomenon, it is always important to rule out reflux and esophagitis by methods previously described before determining that the patient has idiopathic sphincter dysfunction.

ASSOCIATION WITH DIFFUSE ESOPHAGEAL SPASM. Hypertension and poor relaxation of the lower esophageal sphincter have been described in patients with symptomatic idiopathic diffuse esophageal spasm (SIDES).[68] A recent paper, however, indicates that most patients with SIDES do not have lower esophageal sphincter dysfunction[69] (Fig. 9–6). There are certain patients in whom both SIDES and LES dysfunction do occur. Muscular hypertrophy of the esophagus has been described in some of these patients.[70]

IDIOPATHIC LES DYSFUNCTION. Isolated dysfunction of the LES with sphincter hypertension, hypercontraction, or poor relaxation has been described and probably represents a separate clinical entity.[71] The presence of gastroesophageal reflux must be excluded before this diagnosis can be entertained.

ASSOCIATION WITH DIVERTICULA. Diverticula of the esophagus occur infrequently and are generally of unknown etiology. They may result from the forceful esophageal contractile activity necessary to overcome LES outlet obstruction[72] (Fig. 9–7). The disappearance of multiple esophageal diverticula following treatment of reflux esophagitis has been reported.[73]

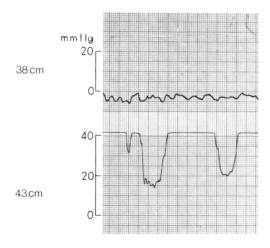

Figure 9-4. LES in achalasia. Resting pressure is high (over 40 mm Hg). Relaxation is incomplete.

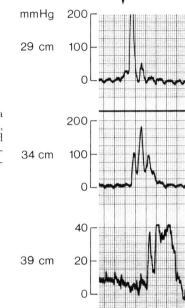

Figure 9-5.   Esophageal body and LES in a patient with gastroesophageal reflux. At 39 cm, the LES is hypotensive and relaxes normally and hypercontracts following a swallow. The peristaltic wave is hypertensive, probably because of irritation.

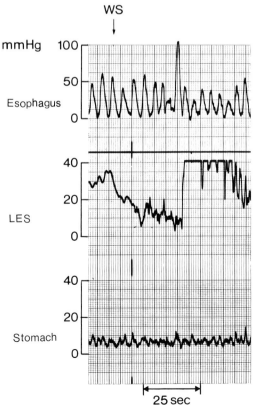

Figure 9-6.   LES in SIDES. The middle channel shows a normal resting pressure gradient. Relaxation is normal. In some patients with SIDES, however, LES dysfunction does occur. (WS, wet swallow.)

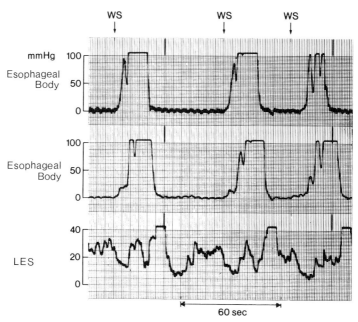

Figure 9-7.   Esophageal body and LES abnormalities in a patient with an epiphrenic diverticulum. Incoordination between LES relaxation and the broad hypertensive oncoming wave is present. Premature sphincter contraction occurs. (*WS*, wet swallow.)

Dysphagia is the distinguishing feature of the "hypertensive LES syndrome," since the LES presents a barrier to the passage of the food bolus as it moves from esophagus to stomach. Patients sense food "sticking" at the lower end of the sternum and may have to wash solids down by drinking large quantities of liquids in order to effect passage. Pain with swallowing (odynophagia), as well as chest pain from forceful nonpropulsive esophageal contractions may also be present.

EVALUATION

MANOMETRY.   LESP is usually elevated, and relaxation to gastric base line may not be complete following swallows. As a result, a pressure gradient between the sphincter and gastric base line persists (Fig. 9–3). Poor coordination with the oncoming esophageal peristaltic wave may also be present, so that the bolus arrives at the sphincter when it is not relaxed. Such functional abnormalities of the LES may be fairly constant or may occur only intermittently.

pH STUDIES.   pH studies should be performed in these patients, since on occasion a hypertensive, poorly relaxing sphincter may be the result of gastroesophageal reflux. The mechanism is presumed to involve local irritation of sphincteric tissue.

ACID PERFUSION STUDIES.   These studies may demonstrate esophageal irritability to acid perfusion if the LES abnormalities are due to gastroesophageal reflux.

ENDOSCOPY AND BIOPSY.   Endoscopy should be performed to exclude the presence of encroaching structural lesions and to determine whether or not esophagitis is present.

RADIOGRAPHIC STUDIES.   Radiography may initially suggest the correct diagnosis. A picture of diffuse esophageal spasm or one of nonpropulsive activity may be noted at the time of radiography. Some patients with a syndrome of hypertensive lower esophageal sphincter and diffuse spasm may have muscular hypertrophy of the esophagus.[70] Such esophageal muscle thickening may often be seen by radiographic means and may be very helpful in suggesting the proper diagnosis.

TREATMENT

Treatment of these conditions is not uniform. Certainly if gastroesophageal reflux is present, antireflux treatment may be quite beneficial. The other aspects of this syndrome may be treated by bougienage, pneumatic dilatation, or long esophagomyotomy. These therapies are discussed elsewhere in this book.

REFERENCES

1. Castell D. O.: The lower esophageal sphincter. Physiologic and clinical aspects. Ann. Intern. Med., 83:390–401, 1975.
2. Pope C. E. 2nd: Pathophysiology and diagnosis of reflux esophagitis. Gastroenterology, 70:445–454, 1976.
3. Clarke S. D., Penry J. B., Ward P.: Oesophageal reflux after abdominal vagotomy. Lancet, 2:824–826, 1965.
4. Crispin J. S., McIver D. K., Lind J. G.: Manometric study of the effect of vagotomy on the gastroesophageal sphincter. Can. J. Surg., 10:299–303, 1967.
5. Carveth S. W., Schlegel J. F., Code C. F., Ellis F. H.: Esophageal motility after vagotomy, phrenicotomy, myotomy and myomectomy in dogs. Surg. Gynecol. Obstet., 114:31–42, 1962.
6. Matarazzo S. A., Snape W. J., Ryan J. P., Cohen S.: Relationship of cervical and abdominal vagal activity to lower esophageal sphincter function. Gastroenterology, 71:999–1003, 1976.
7. Mann C. V., Hardcastle J. D.: The effect of vagotomy on the human gastroesophageal sphincter. Gut, 9:688–695, 1968.
8. Blackman A. H., Rakatansky H., Nasrullah M., Thayer W. R.: Transabdominal vagectomy and lower esophageal function. Arch. Surg., 102:6–8, 1971.
9. Mazur J. M., Skinner D. B., Jones E. L., et al.: Effect of transabdominal vagotomy on the human gastroesophageal sphincter. Surgery, 73:818–822, 1973.
10. Lind J. F., Crispin J. S., McIver D. K.: The effect of atropine on the gastroesophageal sphincter. J. Physiol. Pharmacol., 46:233–238, 1968.

11. Fisher R. S., Malmud L. S., Roberts G. S., Lobis I. F.: The lower esophageal sphincter as a barrier to gastroesophageal reflux. Gastroenterology, 72:19–22, 1977.
12. Kelley M. L., Friedland H. I.: Gastroesophageal sphincteric pressures before and after oral anticholinergic drug and placebo administration. Am. J. Dig. Dis., 12:823–833, 1967.
13. Van Thiel D. H., Gavaler J. S., Stremple J.: Lower esophageal sphincter pressure in women using sequential oral contraceptives. Gastroenterology, 71:232–234, 1976.
14. Schulze K., Christensen J.: Lower sphincter of the opossum esophagus in pseudo-pregnancy. Gastroenterology, 73:1082–1085, 1977.
15. Mandelstam P., Siegel C. I., Lieber A. et al.: The swallowing disorder in patients with diabetic neuropathy-gastroenteropathy. Gastroenterology, 56:1–11, 1969.
16. Hollis J. B., Castell D. O., Braddom R. L.: Esophageal function in diabetes mellitus and its relation to peripheral neuropathy. Gastroenterology, 73:1098–1102, 1977.
17. Nebel O. T., Castell D. O.: Lower esophageal sphincter changes after food ingestion. Gastroenterology, 63:778–783, 1972.
18. Wright L. E., Castell D. O.: The adverse effect of chocolate on lower esophageal sphincter pressure. Am. J. Dig. Dis., 20:703–707, 1975.
19. Dennish G. W., Castell D. O.: Inhibitory effect of smoking on the lower esophageal sphincter. N. Engl. J. Med., 284:1136–1137, 1971.
20. Castell D. O.: Changes in lower esophageal sphincter pressure during insulin-induced hypoglycemia. Gastroenterology, 61:10–15, 1971.
21. Higgs R. H., Smyth R. D., Castell D. O.: Gastric alkalinization: effect on lower esophageal sphincter pressure and serum gastrin. N. Engl. J. Med., 291:486–490, 1974.
22. Lataste L., Gouthier F.: LES reflux oesophagiens apres gastrectomies distales. Presse Méd., 75:1025–1028, 1967.
23. Lipschutz W., Cohen S.: Physiologic determinants of lower esophageal sphincter function. Gastroenterology, 61:16–24, 1971.
24. Kline M. M., McCallum R. W., Curry N., Sturdevant R. A. L.: Effect of gastric alkalinization on lower esophageal sphincter pressure and serum gastrin. Gastroenterology, 68:1137–1139, 1975.
25. Farrell R. L., Castell D. O., McGuigan J. E.: Measurements and comparisons of lower esophageal sphincter pressures and serum gastrin levels in patients with gastroestophageal reflux. Gastroenterology, 67:415–422, 1974.
26. Dodds W. J., Hogan W. J., Miller W. N., Barreras R. F., Arndorfer R. C., Steff J. J.: Relationship between serum gastrin concentration and lower esophageal sphincter pressure. Am. J. Dig. Dis., 20:201–207, 1975.
27. Isenberg J., Csendes A., Walsh J. H.: Resting and pentagastrin-stimulated gastro-esophageal sphincter pressure in patients with Zollinger-Ellison syndrome. Gastroenterology, 61:655–658, 1971.
28. Farrell R. L., Nebel O. T., McGuire A. T., Castell D. O.: The abnormal lower oesophageal sphincter in pernicious anemia. Gut, 14:767–772, 1973.
29. Cohen S., Booth G. H.: Gastric acid secretion and lower esophageal sphincter pressure in response to coffee and caffeine. N. Engl. J. Med., 293:897–899, 1975.
30. Neuhauser E. B. D., Berenberg W.: Cardio-esophageal relaxation as a cause of vomiting in infants. Radiology, 48:480–483, 1947.
31. Gryboski J. D., Thayer W. R., Spiro H. M.: Esophageal motility in infants and children. Pediatrics, 31:382–395, 1963.
32. Moroz S. P., Espinoza J., Cumming W. A., Diamant N. E.: Lower esophageal sphincter function in children with and without gastroesophageal reflux. Gastroenterology, 71:236–241, 1976.
33. Nagler R., Spiro H. M.: Heartburn in late pregnancy. Manometric studies of esophageal motor function. J. Clin. Invest., 40:954–970, 1961.
34. Lind J. F., Smith A. M., McIver D. K., Coopland A. T., Crispin J. S.: Heartburn in pregnancy — a manometric study. Can. Med. Assoc. J., 98:571–574, 1968.
35. VanThiel D. H., Gavaler J. S., Joshi S. N., Sara R. K., Stremple J.: Heartburn of pregnancy. Gastroenterology, 72:666–668, 1977.

36. Simpson J. A., Conn H. O.: Role of ascites in gastroesophageal reflux with comments on the pathogenesis of bleeding esophageal varices. Gastroenterology, 55:17–25, 1968.
37. Van Thiel D. H., Stremple J. F.: Lower esophageal sphincter pressure in cirrhotic men with ascites: before and after diuresis. Gastroenterology, 72:842–844, 1977.
38. Eastwood G. L., Castell D. O., Higgs R. H.: Experimental esophagitis in cats impairs lower esophageal sphincter pressure. Gastroenterology, 69:146–153, 1975.
39. Orlando R. C., Bozymski E. M.: Heartburn in pernicious anemia—a consequence of bile reflux. N. Engl. J. Med., 289:522–523, 1973.
40. Cohen S., Harris L. D.: Does hiatus hernia affect competence of the gastroesophageal sphincter? N. Engl. J. Med., 284:1053–1056, 1971.
41. Code C. F., Kelley M. L., Schegel J. F., Olsen A. M.: Detection of hiatal hernia during esophageal motility tests. Gastroenterology, 43:521–531, 1962.
42. Affolter H.: Pressure characteristics of reflux esophagitis. Helv. Med. Acta, 33:395–402, 1966.
43. Ramirez J., Guarner V., Pazmino F.: Alterations in motility of the esophagus in peptic esophagitis. Am. J. Proctol., 19:67–73, 1968.
44. Hunt P. S., Connell A. M., Smiley T. B.: The cricopharyngeal sphincter in gastric reflux. Gut, 11:303–306, 1970.
45. Berts L. E., Winans C. S.: Lower esophageal sphincter function does not determine resting upper esophageal sphincter pressure. Am. J. Dig. Dis., 22:877–880, 1977.
46. Brand D. L., Martin D., Pope C. E. 2nd: Esophageal manometrics in patients with angina-like chest pain. Am. J. Dig. Dis., 22:300–304, 1977.
47. Iverson L. I. G., May I. A., Samson P. C.: Pulmonary complications in benign esophageal disease. Am. J. Surg., 126:223–228, 1973.
48. Bennett J. R.: The physician's problem. Gut, 14:246–249, 1973.
49. Haddad J. K.: Relation of gastroesophageal reflux to yield sphincter pressures. Gastroenterology, 58:175–184, 1970.
50. Atkinson M., VanGelder A.: Esophageal intraluminal pH recording in the assessment of gastroesophageal reflux and its consequences. Am. J. Dig. Dis., 22:365–370, 1977.
51. Spencer J.: Prolonged pH recording in the study of gastroesophageal reflux. Br. J. Surg., 56:912–914, 1969.
52. Lichter I.: Measurement of gastroesophageal reflux: its significance in hiatus hernia. Br. J. Surg., 61:253–258, 1974.
53. Ismail-Beigi F., Pope C. E. 2nd: Distribution of the histologic changes of gastroesophageal reflux in the distal esophagus. Gastroenterology, 66:1109–1113, 1974.
54. Ismail-Beigi F., Horton P. F., Pope C. E. 2nd: Histologic consequences of gastroesophageal reflux in man. Gastroenterology, 58:163–174, 1970.
55. Seefeld U., Krejs G. S., Siebenmann R. E., Blum A. L.: Esophageal histology in gastroesophageal reflux. Morphologic findings in suction biopsies. Am. J. Dig. Dis., 22:956–964, 1977.
56. Benz L. J., Hootkin L. A., Margulies S., Donner M. W., Cauthorne R. T., Hendrix T. R.: A comparison of clinical measurements of gastroesophageal reflux. Gastroenterology, 62:1–5, 1972.
57. Fisher R. S., Malmud L. S., Roberts G. S., Lobis I. F.: Gastroesophageal (GE) scintiscanning to detect and quantitate GE reflux. Gastroenterology, 70:301–313, 1976.
58. Booth D. J., Kemmerer W. T., Skinner D. B.: Acid clearing from the distal esophagus. Arch. Surg., 96:731–734, 1968.
59. Stancin C., Bennett J. R.: Oesophageal acid clearing: one factor in the production of reflux oesophagitis. Gut, 15:852–857, 1974.
60. Butterfield D. G., Struthers J. E., Showalter J. P.: A test of gastroesophageal sphincter competence. The common cavity test. Am. J. Dig. Dis., 17:415–421, 1972.
61. Salter R. H.: Lower oesophageal sphincter therapeutic implications. Lancet, 1:347–349, 1974.

62. Farrell R. L., Roling G. T., Castell D. O.: Stimulation of the incompetent lower esophageal sphincter. A possible advance in therapy of heartburn. Am. J. Dig. Dis., 18:646–650, 1973.
63. Farrell R. L., Roling G. T., Castell D. O.: Cholinergic therapy of chronic heartburn. A controlled trial. Ann. Intern. Med., 80:573–576, 1974.
64. Miller W. N., Ganeshopper K. P., Dodds W. J., Hogan W. J., Barreras R. F., Arndorfer R. C.: Effect of bethanechol on gastroesophageal reflux. Am. J. Dig. Dis., 22:230–234, 1977.
65. Behar J., Biancani P.: Effect of oral metoclopramide on gastroesophageal reflux in the post-cibal state. Gastroenterology, 70:331–335, 1976.
66. Freeland G. R., Higgs R. H., Castell D. O.: Lower esophageal sphincter response to oral administration of cimetidine in normal subjects. Gastroenterology, 72:28–30, 1977.
67. Behar J., Brand D. L., Brown F. C., Castell D. O., Cohen S., Crossby R. J., Pope C. E. 2nd, Winans C. S.: Cimetidine in the treatment of symptomatic gastroesophageal reflux. A double blind controlled trial. Gastroenterology, 74:441–448, 1978.
68. Ellis F. H. Jr., Code C. F., Olsen A. M.: Long esophagomyotomy for diffuse spasm of the esophagus and hypertensive gastroesophageal sphincter. Surgery, 48:155–169, 1960.
69. DiMarino A. J., Cohen S.: Characteristics of lower esophageal sphincter function in symptomatic diffuse esophageal spasm. Gastroenterology, 66:1–6, 1974.
70. Westgaard T., Keats T. E.: Diffuse spasm and muscular hypertrophy of the lower esophagus. Radiology, 90:1001–1005, 1968.
71. Garrett J. M.: Gastroesophageal hypercontracting sphincter. J. A. M. A., 208:992–998, 1969.
72. Cross F.: Esophageal diverticula-related neuromuscular problems. Ann. Otol., 77:914–926, 1968.
73. Bender M. K., Haddad J. K.: Disappearance of multiple esophageal diverticula following treatment of esophagitis. Gastrointest. Endoscopy, 20:19–22, 1973.

CHAPTER 10

THE EFFECTS OF SURGERY ON ESOPHAGEAL FUNCTION

A major role of the esophageal motility study is to evaluate objectively the pathophysiology of primary and secondary motor disorders of the esophagus. In recent years the motility study has quantified the therapeutic and adverse effects of surgery on the esophagus. Its use has permitted a more rational approach to the surgical management of the patient with disordered swallowing. The present chapter will discuss the beneficial and detrimental effects of surgery on esophageal motor function.

THE EFFECTS OF SURGERY ON THE UPPER ESOPHAGEAL SPHINCTER (UES)

Two aspects of the physiologic effect of surgery on the pharyngoesophageal sphincter will be examined: the therapeutic effects and the adverse effects (Table 10–1).

THERAPEUTIC EFFECTS

The two most frequent operations performed on the upper esophageal sphincter are pharyngoesophageal diverticulectomy and cricopharyngeal (UES) myotomy. While much has been written on the effects of surgery on the function of the lower esophageal sphincter LES), very few reports discuss the influence of surgery on UES motor function.

Diverticulectomy. Cricopharyngeal (Zenker's) diverticulectomy has been performed for many years. The results of this operation are most satisfying.[1] Manometrically, no change is noted in the length

TABLE 10–1.   *Effects of Surgery on the Esophagus*

EFFECTS OF SURGERY ON THE UPPER ESOPHAGEAL SPHINCTER (UES)
    Therapeutic Effects
        Diverticulectomy
        Cricopharyngeal myotomy
    Adverse Effects
        Topical anesthesia
        Recurrent laryngeal nerve palsy
        Laryngectomy
        Tracheostomy

EFFECTS OF SURGERY ON THE LOWER ESOPHAGEAL SPHINCTER (LES)
AND ON THE ESOPHAGEAL BODY
    Therapeutic Effects
        Hiatal hernia repair
            a. Simple repair
                Anatomic repair
                Hill posterior gastropexy
                Nissen fundoplication
                Belsey repair
            b. Repair for the short and/or strictured esophagus
                Collis gastroplasty
                Thal fundic patch repair
                Intrathoracic fundoplication
        Myotomy of the distal esophagus and LES
            a. Modified Heller myotomy for achalasia
            b. Long esophageal myotomy for symptomatic idiopathic
               diffuse esophageal spasm

    Adverse Effects
        Vagotomy
            Experimental vagotomy
            Clinical vagotomy
        Transection of the esophagus
        Repair of esophageal atresia and tracheoesophageal fistula
        Transection and diversion
        Response to obstruction

and basal pressure of the sphincter. Coordination and relaxation of the UES remain normal as well.[2]

Cricopharyngeal Myotomy.   Cricopharyngeal (UES) myotomy has been reported in the recent literature in more than 230 patients.[3] This operation is performed for the smaller-sized pharyngoesophageal diverticula and for primary or secondary oropharyngeal dysphagia. Cricopharyngeal myotomy simply abolishes the pressure gradient that exists between the pharynx and the esophagus, thus permitting an easier transit through the region of the UES. Pre-existent defects in coordination persist after surgery.

Manometric evaluation before and after myotomy for pharyngoesophageal diverticulum reveals a significant reduction of the resting pressure in the proximal esophageal sphincter. The manometric length of the sphincter is also diminished. These changes remain the same from 7 to 24 months after surgery. The abnormal temporal

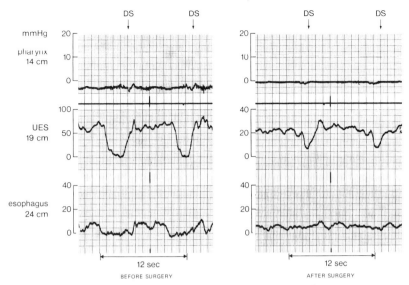

Figure 10-1. UES function before and after cricopharyngeal myotomy in a patient with oculopharyngeal muscular dystrophy. Before surgery pharyngeal contractions are barely visible and are not coordinated with UES relaxation. After surgery, the motility disturbance persists, but the resting pressure in the UES is reduced. (*DS*, dry swallow.)

relationship between pharyngoesophageal sphincter relaxation and pharyngeal contraction (present in 14 to 90 percent of the swallows) remains after surgery.[4]

Similar observations were recently reported following UES myotomy in patients with oropharyngeal dysphagia secondary to oculopharyngeal muscular dystrophy.[5] UES myotomy in 11 patients produced marked relief of the dysphagia by lowering the sphincter pressure by approximately 50 percent. The very weak pharyngeal contractions remained unchanged (Fig. 10–1).

Controversy still exists over the response of the UES to gastroesophageal reflux. Oropharyngeal dysphagia is reported to be present in as many as 50 percent of patients with reflux. Twenty percent of the group have severe oropharyngeal dysphagia, and 10 percent will not respond to adequate correction of the reflux.[6, 7] Manometric studies show premature contraction of the UES relative to the pharyngeal contraction. Cricopharyngeal myotomy may be performed in those patients who are not improved by antireflux surgery. The myotomy is effective in relieving symptoms and in lowering UES pressure, although the UES coordination defect persists. Because of the threat of aspiration of gastroduodenal contents, UES myotomy should only be considered in patients whose underlying LES hypotension and gastroesophageal reflux have been treated.

Any procedure that interrupts the neuromuscular and vascular integrity of the pharyngoesophageal junction may have an adverse effect on UES motor function.

Topical Anesthesia.   Topical anesthesia of the pharynx produces incoordination of the UES. It creates a prolonged pharyngeal contraction while shortening the relaxation phase of the UES.[8] The medullary swallowing center is dependent on continuous sensory information about bolus position during the act of deglutition. This appears to be lost with local anesthesia.

Recurrent Laryngeal Nerve Palsy.   Since the motor innervation of the upper sphincter area is probably vagal in origin, any interruption of the local fibers may produce UES dysfunction. Henderson reported 18 patients with recurrent laryngeal nerve palsy who all had symptoms of oropharyngeal dysphagia. The manometric abnormalities noted were a loss of pharyngeal cricopharyngeal coordination, with the pharyngeal contraction wave occurring before maximal UES relaxation.[9]

Laryngectomy.   Laryngectomy for treatment of cancer interrupts vagal fibers and transects the most proximal part of the digestive tube. Laryngectomy patients have lower resting and contraction pressure of the upper sphincter in comparison to controls. A lower degree of UES pharyngeal coordination and a lower incidence of complete UES relaxation are also noted[10, 11, 12] (Fig. 10–2). In one experimental study that followed supraglottic laryngectomy, electromyography showed spastic contractions of the cricopharyngeus without normal inhibitory activity of the muscle. Cricopharyngeal myotomy returned the inhibition phase to normal.[13] Schobinger, in 42 patients studied after radical neck dissection and after laryngectomy, observed 10 patients in whom spastic contractions of the cricopharyngeus were identified.[12]

Winans studied the correlations of the quality of alaryngeal voice with UES pressure.[14] Those patients with high UES pressure after laryngectomy had poor esophageal speech. Patients with lower UES resting pressure were better able to develop high quality alaryngeal speech.

Tracheostomy.   Patients who undergo tracheostomy may suffer from oropharyngeal dysphagia. The mechanism involved seems to be a limited relaxation of the UES by direct inhibition of the hypomandibular complex.[15] Cicatricial scarring precludes laryngeal elevation with swallows. This leads to ineffectual pharyngeal contraction and poor UES relaxation.

In summary, primary sphincteric abnormalities, devascularization, nerve interruption, laryngeal or pharyngeal transection, muscle fixation by various surgical procedures, and tracheostomy may result in oropharyngeal dysphagia secondary to UES dysfunction., Crico-

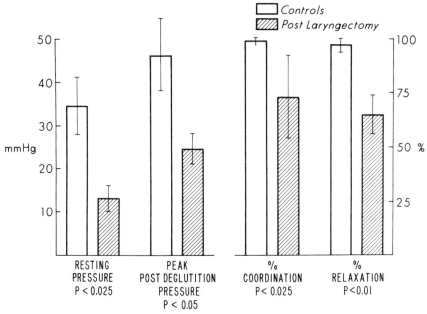

Figure 10-2. UES function after laryngectomy. Significant motor abnormalities are observed in the UES after this procedure. Reprinted from Duranceau A., Jamieson G., Hurwitz A. L., Jones R. S., Postlethwait R. W.: Alteration in esophageal motility after laryngectomy. Am. J. Surg., 131:30–35, 1976 (by permission).

pharyngeal myotomy may be of value in bringing relief to these patients by lowering the UES resting pressure. Most of the evidence suggests unaltered UES motor dysfunction after myotomy.

THE EFFECTS OF SURGERY ON THE LOWER ESOPHAGEAL SPHINCTER (LES) AND ON THE ESOPHAGEAL BODY

Since the LES and the body of the esophagus are two closely related units, the functional results of surgery on both areas will be considered together (Table 10–1).

THERAPEUTIC EFFECTS

Therapeutic surgical procedures have measurable effects on the motility of the gastroesophageal junction and of the esophageal body. These procedures include a variety of hiatal hernia repairs, the short myotomy for achalasia, and the long myotomy for symptomatic idiopathic diffuse esophageal spasm (SIDES).

Hiatal Hernia Repair

Hypotension of the lower esophageal sphincter is common in the presence of reflux symptoms and esophagitis.[16, 17, 18] The pathogenesis of LES hypotension is not known (see Chapter 9). It may be a primary process or secondary to the reflux injury. When esophagitis is induced experimentally with acid and bile, the tone of the LES declines, and secondary abnormalities in peristalsis occur. Disappearance of the esophagitis is followed by a progressive return to normal LES tone.[19, 20] Impaired esophageal stripping waves appear in patients with symptoms of reflux when the esophagus is perfused with acid.[21] Olsen and Henderson reported a high correlation between the severity of abnormal motor activity and the damage caused to the esophagus by gastroesophageal reflux.[22, 23]

The effects on the esophagus following surgical hiatal hernia repair are measurable both in terms of pressure change and in terms of the incidence of disordered esophageal motor activity. The goal of surgical correction of hiatal hernia is to create a sufficient length of intra-abdominal esophagus and to restore normal resting tone to the hypotensive LES. Elimination of reflux should result from a good repair. Tables 10–2 and 10–3 depict the various surgical repairs used at present, with their respective morbidities, mortalities, and physiologic effects on the esophagus.

Anatomic Hiatal Hernia Repair.   The anatomic repair proposed by Allison has been shown experimentally to restore LES pressure.[24, 25] However, no improvement in the ability of the sphincter to contract is observed.[26] Simple anatomic correction of a hiatal hernia with this method leads to a radiologically detected recurrence rate of 49 percent for the sliding hernia and a 33 percent recurrence rate for the paraesophageal hernia.[27]

Collis devised an abdominothoracic approach for an anatomic repair of hiatal hernias. It was observed that if the patient had no preoperative LES tone, then no tone was found postoperatively. In the body of the esophagus, peristalsis showed an increased amplitude after surgery, possibly resulting in better esophageal clearance. The results of this procedure reported in 200 patients showed persistence of moderate reflux in 10 percent of the patients, free reflux in 9 percent of the group, and a 2.5 percent incidence of recurrent hernias.[28, 29]

Hill Posterior Gastropexy.   The Hill procedure "calibrates" the cardia and anchors the lesser curvature of the stomach to the median arcuate ligament, creating a posterior gastropexy. A number of studies have shown that significantly higher LES pressures are obtained by such a hiatal hernia repair.[30-33] Hill recently updated his data using intraoperative manometry. In 154 patients, LESP was calibrated during the operation to a level of 50 to 55 mm Hg. In this group of patients the mean preoperative LESP was 6.9 mm Hg. After surgery, mean resting LESP was 19.1 mm Hg.[34]

TABLE 10–2. *Standard Repair*

OPERATION	MORBIDITY	MORTALITY	MANOMETRIC AND pH RESPONSE	RECURRENCE RATE		
				SYMPTOMS	RADIOLOGICAL	pH
ALLISON REPAIR	– DIAPHRAGMATIC INCISIONAL HERNIA	0.3%	LES PRESSURE ↑ pH _____	20 – 31%	32 – 49%	——
COLLIS PLASTIC REPAIR	——	SLIDING 1.5% PARAESOPHAGEAL 5.0%	LES PRESSURE ↑ pH: IMPROVED	21 – 24%	2.5%	5%
POSTERIOR GASTROPEXY (HILL REPAIR)	– DYSPHAGIA – ARTERIAL INJURY TO CELIAC AXIS – VAGAL TRAUMA – ESOPHAGEAL PERFORATION – ESOPHAGEAL FISTULA	0.3%	LES PRESSURE ↑ pH: IMPROVED	3 – 10% 17% IF STRICTURE AND/OR SHORT ESOPHAGUS	6 – 7%	6 – 10% STANDARD TEST 20% 24 HR. TEST 27%
PARTIAL FUNDOPLICATION (BELSEY REPAIR)	– ESOPHAGEAL PERFORATION OR NECROSIS – VAGAL NERVE AND ARTERIAL BRANCHES INJURY – DYSPHAGIA: RARE – GAS BLOAT	1%	LES PRESSURE ↑ pH: IMPROVED	10 – 20% 45–50% IF STRICTURE AND/OR SHORT ESOPHAGUS	7 – 20%	STANDARD TEST 40% 24 HR. TEST 54%
TOTAL FUNDOPLICATION (NISSEN REPAIR)	– DYSPHAGIA – GAS BLOAT: EARLY 10–55% LATE 12–15% – DEHISCENCE OR SLIPPING OF PLICATION – PERFORATION OF THE ESOPHAGUS – SUBPHRENIC ABCESS – INCIDENTAL SPLENECTOMY 7–18%	1–1.2%	LES PRESSURE ↑ pH: IMPROVED	0 – 10%	0 – 5%	STANDARD TEST 0% 24 HR. TEST 0%

Some studies suggest a return to normal physiologic function of the sphincter after the Hill repair.[30-32] Other reports, however, show that neural integrity of the LES is not restored with the creation of an antireflux barrier.[26] One study reported that esophageal stricture disappeared following posterior gastropexy in which LES pressure was restored to normal.[31]

An overall hiatal hernia recurrence rate of 3 to 10 percent is reported after the Hill repair.[30, 35] In the group of patients who had intraoperative manometric documentation, a single recurrence has been reported.

Nissen Fundoplication.   In the Nissen fundoplication, a gastric fundic wrap of 360 degrees encircles the distal esophagus, creating an effective barrier to reflux.[36] A number of experimental studies have shown that significantly higher pressures are created in the LES zone by such a repair[37-41] (Fig. 10–3 A and B). In addition, an increase in positive intragastric pressure produces a further increase in the high pressure zone created by the procedure. Most studies

TABLE 10-3. *Repair for Short and/or Strictured Esophagus*

OPERATION	MORBIDITY	MORTALITY	MANOMETRIC AND pH RESPONSE	RECURRENCE RATE		
				CLINICAL	RADIOLOGICAL	pH
COLLIS GASTROPLASTY WITH PARTIAL FUNDOPLICATION	– FUNCTIONAL OBSTRUCTION – SPLEEN INJURY – GASTROCUTANEOUS FISTULA – ISCHEMIC NECROSIS OF THE ESOPHAGUS – ESOPHAGEAL PERFORATION – GASTROPLASTY TUBE LEAK	0–2.5%	– LES PRESSURE ↑ IMPROVED – pH IMPROVED – ESOPHAGEAL BODY FUNCTION IMPROVED	6–25%	0–2.5%	30–46%
COLLIS GASTROPLASTY WITH TOTAL FUNDOPLICATION	– FUNCTIONAL OBSTRUCTION – DELAYED EMPTYING – GAS BLOAT – ESOPHAGEAL PERFORATION – GASTROPLASTY TUBE NECROSIS – SHORT GASTRIC VESSEL BLEEDING – GASTROPLASTY TUBE LEAK	0–3.3%	– LES PRESSURE ↑ IMPROVED – pH IMPROVED – ESOPHAGEAL BODY FUNCTION IMPROVED	0%	0.3%	0–3.3%
INTRATHORACIC NISSEN FUNDOPLICATION	– INCISIONAL HERNIA THROUGH DIAPHRAGM AND HIATUS – ESOPHAGEAL LEAK – ULCER AND HEMORRAGE FROM SUPRADIAPHRAGMATIC STOMACH – PAIN OF INCARCERATED HERNIA	UNDETERMINED	– HIGH PRESSURE ZONE WITHOUT SPHINCTER FUNCTION	—	—	FREE REFLUX IF INCOMPLETE INTRATHORACIC FUNDOPLICATION
THAL FUNDIC PATCH REPAIR	– SAME AS ABOVE	1–5%	– HIGH PRESSURE ZONE WITHOUT SPHINCTER FUNCTION	13–27%	—	FREE REFLUX IF INCOMPLETE INTRATHORACIC FUNDOPLICATION

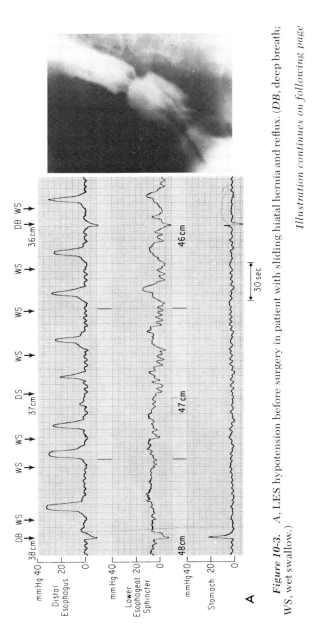

Figure 10-3. A, LES hypotension before surgery in patient with sliding hiatal hernia and reflux. (*DB*, deep breath; *WS*, wet swallow.)

Illustration continues on following page

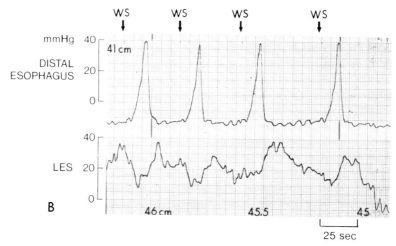

Figure 10-3. Continued. B, Same patient after a Nissen fundoplication. The LESP is restored, although relaxation of the LES is incomplete after swallowing.

conclude that the LES-gastric gradient is due to a simple mechanical effect of the gastric musculature wrapped around the distal esophagus.[42, 43] Siewert proposes that fundoplication yields desirable results only in the incompetent sphincter. He feels that the fundus wrap created from the muscular wall adjacent to the cardia is subjected to myogenic and hormonal regulation similar to that of the LES.[44]

Of all hiatal hernia repairs, the Nissen fundoplication creates the greatest increase in LES pressure and is the most effective in preventing reflux as determined by pH and scintiscanning studies.[39, 41, 45] Even an incomplete fundoplication, with as much as a 1 cm gap, leaves a significant residual sphincter-to-stomach gradient after relaxation of the LES.[43] The high pressure zone created by a Nissen repair may lead to impaired esophageal emptying if poor peristalsis is present in the esophageal body. Therefore this operation is not suggested as an antireflux procedure in patients with impaired peristalsis, scleroderma, or after myotomy for achalasia.[33, 44]

A recurrence rate of 0 to 10 percent is reported with the Nissen fundoplication. The major morbidity associated with this repair is the "gas-bloat" syndrome (inability to belch) that occurs in 12 to 50 percent of the cases. Trauma to the spleen necessitating incidental splenectomy is also a reported complication.[38, 41, 46]

Belsey Repair.   The Belsey Mark IV repair creates a *partial* anterolateral fundoplication of the stomach on the distal esophagus, with fixation under the diaphragm. This procedure ensures that the distal esophagus and LES are maintained in an intra-abdominal position.

When the LES is properly repositioned by this procedure, an adequate resting LESP is created[47] (Fig. 10–4). In one study, a normal LES adaptive response to abdominal compression and to humoral

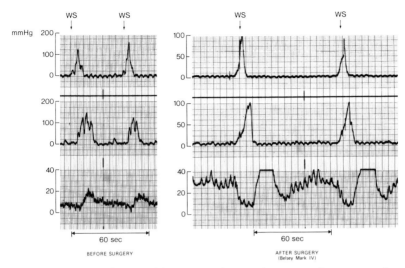

Figure 10-4.   LES function following a Belsey Mark IV repair for gastroesophageal reflux. Following surgery the hypotensive LES pressure is restored to normal. The high pressure zone relaxes normally with swallowing. (WS, wet swallow.)

stimulation was described following the Belsey Mark IV repair.[32] Two other studies, however, show that neurohumoral integrity is not restored after surgery.[48, 49] Normal physiologic LES function following surgical repair has not been firmly established.

If extensive reflux-induced damage has occurred, and the Belsey repair is performed on a shortened scarred esophagus, the partial plication may slide into the thorax. An intrathoracic Belsey plication does not create an adequate pressure zone, and free reflux occurs. By contrast, full Nissen fundoplication around the distal esophagus will prevent subsequent damage by reflux, even if the repair remains intrathoracic or slides into the chest.

The Belsey hiatal hernia repair has a recurrence rate of 12 percent after a 3 year interval. After a 10 year follow-up period, the recurrence rate increases to nearly 15 percent. If a Mark IV correction is performed on a shortened or strictured esophagus, there is a 45 percent recurrence rate.[50]

Collis Gastroplasty.   When the hiatal hernia is irreducible because of esophageal shortening, thickening, or stricture, standard repairs will lead to an unacceptably high recurrence rate of gastroesophageal reflux. In these special circumstances, the Collis gastroplasty may be used. In this operation, a 5 to 6 cm gastric tube is created on the lesser curvature of the stomach. This results in an "elongation" of the esophagus. Partial or total fundoplication of the gastric fundus is then used to enhance the antireflux mechanism. Used in patients with scleroderma, this procedure was found to control reflux satisfactorily.[51] The pressure gradient observed in the gastric tube segment of these patients was 0 to 2 cm H_2O. Controversy still exists regarding measurement accuracy in the gastric tube of the gastroplasty. Intraoperative manometric studies performed with microtransducers document high resting pressures in the tube when a partial fundoplication of the Belsey type is added.[52] The addition of a Nissen fundoplication to the Collis gastroplasty also elevates the postoperative pressure significantly.[53]

Following gastroplasty and partial fundoplication, disordered motor activity in the body of the esophagus is diminished by 2.6 percent. With gastroplasty and a full fundoplication, these abnormalities are diminished by 17.5 percent. Presumably this reduction in esophageal body motility disturbance is the result of a decrease in gastroesophageal reflux.

The radiologic recurrence rate after a gastroplasty with partial fundoplication is reported to be 2.5 percent. With a full fundoplication the hernia will recur in 0.3 percent of the patients.

Intrathoracic Nissen Fundoplication and Thal Fundic Patch Repair. An alternative to the Collis gastroplasty is the total Nissen fundoplication, which may be left in the chest in the presence of a short esophagus. When an established stricture is present, the Thal repair may also be used. In the Thal procedure, the stricture is incised and the serosa of the gastric fundus is used to cover the divided esophagus. Thal noted a pressure of 10 to 15 mm Hg in the segment of esophagus enclosed by the stomach.[54] Free reflux occurs when the Thal repair remains above the diaphragm. A complete fundoplication combined with the Thal serosal patch creates an adequate high pressure zone that is effective against reflux. This zone, however, will not relax as a normal sphincter does.[55, 56]

The most frequent complication following the Thal repair is entrapment of abdominal contents between the stomach and the diaphragm. Cases of lethal gastric ulcers in the gastric pouch above the diaphragm have also been reported.[57, 58]

In summary, most surgical procedures correct reflux by restoring a high pressure zone at the gastroesophageal junction. The mechanisms by which such barriers are created still require clarification. Most evidence suggests that the barrier is mechanical. That a "physiologic" sphincter is restored is not proven.

Myotomy of the Distal Esophagus and Distal Sphincter

Modified Heller's Myotomy. The modified Heller's myotomy is the surgical treatment of choice for achalasia (see also Chapter 8). Satisfactory results are obtained in 93 percent of the cases, with a mortality rate of 1 percent.[59]

The therapeutic effects of the modified Heller's operation have been documented both experimentally and clinically. After myotomy is performed in animals with experimentally induced achalasia, marked reduction of the LES pressure is observed. Abnormal LES relaxation persists, and the LES pressure gradient is never completely eliminated. There is no difference in the residual LESP produced by various types of myotomy.[59, 60, 61]

The surgical results of the modified Heller's myotomy are reported in a number of studies. In a group of 18 patients who had undergone myotomy 1 to 9 years previously, no sphincter could be identified manometrically in seven, and there was a residual sphincter in 11. In a second group of patients, manometry was performed before and after surgery. A lower LES resting pressure and a diminished length of the LES were observed postoperatively. A partial high pressure zone was retained in the subhiatal portion of the sphincter, and the authors stated that this was sufficient to prevent significant reflux.[62]

The long-term physiologic effects of myotomy remain the same. A persistent high pressure zone in the sphincter area suggests a return of the sphincteric muscle function by reapproximation of the myotomized segment or by the development of a postoperative stricture.[59] Esophageal body contractions and coordination are not affected by the myotomy, but resting esophageal pressure may be reduced.

Pneumatic dilatation disrupts the LES and distal esophageal muscular fibers. Successful dilatation produces a decrease in the resting pressure within the LES and an increase in the amplitude of contractions in the body of the esophagus. This elevation in the amplitude of contractions correlates with a decrease in the diameter of the esophagus.[63, 64] Pneumatic dilatation gives satisfactory results in 60 percent of the cases with an incidence of perforation of 3 percent.[65, 66]

Satisfactory results in the pneumatic and surgical treatment of achalasia are accompanied by nearly complete abolition of the pressure gradient between the stomach and esophagus (Fig. 10–5). The diameter of the esophagus is usually diminished as well, but this change may be very slow in advanced cases.[64, 67]

If the LES pressure gradient is abolished by a modified Heller's myotomy, gastroesophageal reflux may occur. In one study, 2 percent of the patients who underwent postoperative radiologic studies demonstrated reflux. In this same group, 10 out of 16 patients with poor results showed evidence of damage by reflux esophagitis.[59] Belsey reports an incidence of reflux in 22 percent of patients following myotomy.[68] Two additional studies showed reflux in 18 percent and 30 percent of the patients, respectively.[69, 70]

Collis studied 108 patients who underwent a Heller's cardiomyotomy and who were followed for 4 or more years. Three groups of patients were studied: 53 had a cardiomyotomy alone, 44 had myotomy plus a simple crural repair, and 11 had a formal hiatal hernia

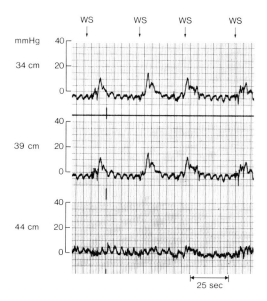

Figure 10-5. Achalasia. LES and esophageal body after a modified Heller's myotomy. Resting esophageal body pressure is normal, and the LES pressure barrier (distal channel) is lost. (WS, wet swallow.)

repair (Collis plastic repair). Thirty-two percent of the first group developed reflux symptoms. When the crural repair was added 46 percent of the second group of patients developed reflux. If a formal hiatal hernia repair was performed, no reflux symptoms occurred.[71]

Since free gastroesophageal reflux is reported in a substantial number of patients following an esophageal myotomy, an antireflux procedure may be contemplated after such a procedure. The antireflux operation must not create a distal high pressure zone that presents an obstacle to the nonfunctioning esophageal body. Well-planned prospective studies are needed to clarify the need for antireflux surgery after myotomy for achalasia.

Long Esophageal Myotomy. Long esophageal myotomy may be performed in patients with severe symptomatic idiopathic diffuse esophageal spasm (SIDES) not responding to conventional medical management. The LES in primary diffuse spasm usually shows normal resting pressure and normal relaxation.[72] If LES function is normal, the myotomy should spare the sphincter. Only the diseased muscle of the organ should be incised. In one study, the effects of long myotomy were reported in five patients with diffuse spasm. A marked diminution of the esophageal body resting and contraction pressures was observed. The underlying motility disturbance was not affected, and proximal esophageal function remained unchanged.[73] In a recent investigation, 10 patients were studied before and after a long myotomy for diffuse spasm. Before surgery, the mean esophageal body pressure was 70 mm Hg; it dropped postoperatively to 20 mm Hg. The LES was left intact and maintained a pressure of 13 mm Hg after surgery, a barrier that was sufficient to prevent reflux in all but one patient.[74] Hurwitz reported a case of epiphrenic diverticulum treated by diverticulectomy and long myotomy. This patient showed excessively high contraction pressures in the esophageal body. Associated LES abnormalities of relaxation and coordination were present. The postoperative pressures in the body of the esophagus were normal[75] (see Fig. 10–6 A, B, and C).

The LES may be damaged or obliterated after this operation, and an antireflux procedure may become necessary. In this respect, one study looked at 34 patients divided into two equal groups. After a long esophageal myotomy, a Belsey procedure was added in the first

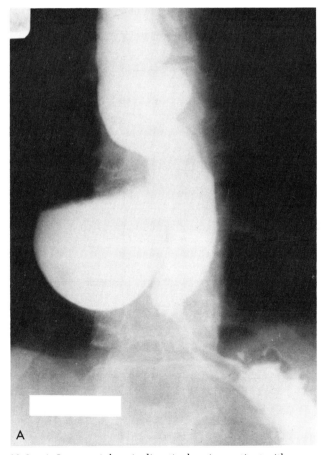

A

Figure 10-6.   A, Large epiphrenic diverticulum in a patient with severe substernal pain.

Illustration continues on following page

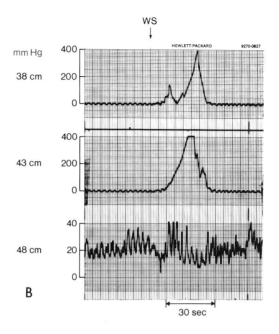

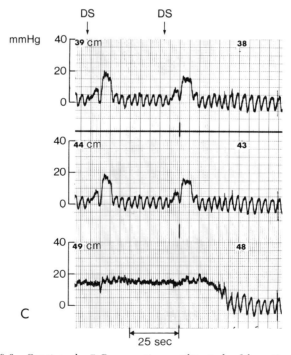

Figure 10-6. Continued. B, Preoperative motility study of the patient whose radiograph appears in *A*. Broad-based, high pressure, nonpropulsive esophageal body waves are seen in conjunction with a poorly relaxing LES (WS, wet swallow.) *C*, Postoperative motility tracing of the same patient after a long esophageal myotomy and diverticulectomy. The esophageal body waves are of normal width and lower amplitude. The distal channel high pressure zone is the result of an antireflux procedure. (*DS*, dry swallow.)

group — 50 percent went on to develop symptomatic reflux. When a Collis gastroplasty coupled with a Belsey fundoplication was performed in the other 17 patients, no symptoms and no reflux occurred.[76]

ADVERSE EFFECTS

Vagotomy

Vagal denervation in any form may adversely influence esophageal motor function. Controversy exists over the effects of different types of vagotomy.

Experimental Vagotomy.   The degree of esophageal motor dysfunction depends on the level of vagotomy. Bilateral electrolytic lesions of the vagal nuclei in animals create an achalasia-like condition of the esophagus, with dilatation, loss of peristalsis, and defective relaxation of the LES.[77] Bilateral supranodosal vagotomy also produces aperistalsis in the body of the esophagus; the LES fails to relax, and the LES resting tone is lowered.[78] Bilateral vagotomy, high on the left and below the recurrent laryngeal nerve on the right, produces loss of peristalsis in the body of the esophagus. The LES initially shows a diminution of both resting tone and contraction. Relaxation is abnormal. After 4 to 8 months, LES function progressively improves.[79] Similar observations were made in monkeys.[80] If distal esophageal vagotomy is performed, a transitory esophageal dilatation with higher resting LES pressure and diminished LES relaxation and contraction occurs.[79] If the esophagus is deprived of all extrinsic innervation, the lower esophagus and LES can still respond to distention. This response probably occurs through wall-transmitted innervation independent of the extrinsic nerve supply.[81]

When complete mucosal denervation is performed by separating mucosa from muscularis throughout the entire esophageal circumference, premature repetitive contractions are seen immediately after surgery, but these return to normal within 3 months. LES function remains normal.[82]

Sympathectomy has no effect on the motor function of the body of the esophagus, and no alterations of LES function are noted.[83]

Clinical Studies on Vagotomy.   Much controversy exists over the effects of vagotomy on esophageal function in man. Earlier studies performed with uninfused catheters showed diminished LES pressure after vagotomy. This was in agreement with radiologic studies that described a high incidence of reflux after various types of vagotomy.[84]

In one study, an abnormal response of the LES to abdominal compression was observed following truncal vagotomy and pyloroplasty.[85] The resting pressure in the sphincter remained normal despite this abnormal response. Another study showed normal postoperative LES function.[86] In a third group of patients, water-filled but nonperfused catheters were used to study 11 patients before and after vagotomy — eight showed a fall in maximal LES pressure after surgery.

Parietal cell vagotomy has been reported to cause a 16 percent incidence of reflux.[87] Recent manometric studies, however, show no significant change in the LES function after this operation.[88, 89]

If patients are studied early after vagotomy a transient drop in sphincter function may be observed; this is not so in patients studied longer after vagotomy.[90]

Thomas and Earlam noted a reduced LES length without alteration of LESP in 28 patients studied 6 to 12 months after a vagotomy and drainage procedure. A shorter length and a sustained reduction in LESP have been noted after vagotomy and gastric resection.[91] Of 10 patients evaluated manometrically after vagotomy and antrectomy, six had normal sphincters and four showed hypotensive sphincters. Cholinergic stimulation of the LES remained intact after the operation.[92]

Transection of the Esophagus

Transection of the esophagus may cause LES dysfunction with a decrease in LES pressure, incomplete LES relaxation, and decreased LES contraction pressure. Transection interrupts the propagation of the primary wave, but secondary waves proceed normally to the stomach. Transection with segmental resection results in an interruption of the primary wave at the site of the anastomosis. Simple dissection does not seem to result in functional abnormalities of peristalsis.[93]

Repair of Esophageal Atresia and Tracheoesophageal Fistula

The motor function of the esophagus after repair of esophageal atresia and tracheoesophageal fistula has been well studied. Most investigators agree on the motor abnormalities observed: a short, normal proximal segment, nonpropulsive activity in the mid-esophagus, and a return toward normal function in the distal esophagus and LES (Fig. 10–7). One study reports an achalasia-like pattern in these patients.[94, 95]

Transection and Diversion

With transection and diversion of the cervical esophagus, 25 percent of the swallows still travel through the transection site into the distal esophagus. Most of these contractions are not peristaltic. When the transection is performed at the thoracic level, contrac-

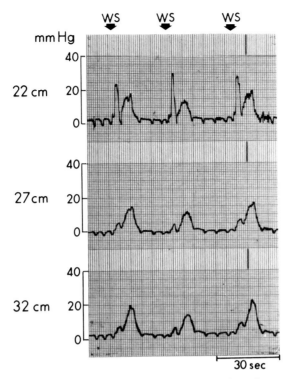

Figure 10-7.   Esophageal motility study following esophageal atresia and tracheo-esophageal fistula repair. A bizarre double-peaked wave is seen in the proximal esophagus. There is no peristalsis in the mid-esophagus. (WS, wet swallow.) Reprinted from Duranceau A., Fisher S. R., Flye M. W., Jones R. S., Postlethwait R. W., Sealy W. C.: Motor function of the esophagus after repair of esophageal atresia and tracheoesophageal fistula. Surgery, 82:116–123, 1977 (by permission of the Editors of Surgery).

tions appear following 65 percent of the swallows, with only 22 percent of the waves being propulsive.[96] In this regard, some contractions may persist in the surgically excluded esophagus.

Response to Obstruction

When mechanical obstruction is present in the esophagus, marked motor dysfunction is observed. Hypotonia of the LES and impairment of LES relaxation and contraction are noted. The contractions of the body of the esophagus are nonpropulsive and generate very high pressures of long duration. Correction of these motor abnormalities has been observed after removal of the obstruction.[97, 98]

FUNCTION OF THE ESOPHAGEAL SUBSTITUTE

An esophageal substitute may be needed to bridge a congenital malformation or to reconstruct the organ following resection for in-

TABLE 10–4.   *Types of Esophageal Substitute*

STOMACH
Interposition
Gastric tube
Free transplant

JEJUNUM AND ILEUM
Interposition
Free transplant

COLON
Interposition
Free transplant

flammatory and malignant conditions. Segments of the digestive tube are usually used, including the stomach, jejunum, and colon. Motor function of the esophageal substitute has been studied both experimentally and clinically (Table 10–4).

Reconstruction with the Stomach

The stomach is most frequently used to restore continuity with the proximal esophageal remnant. Its excellent vascular supply permits a viable esophagogastric anastomosis in the chest or in the neck. The motor function of the interposed stomach has been described; the resting intragastric pressure is positive, even in an intrathoracic position, and falls gradually after a two year period (Fig.

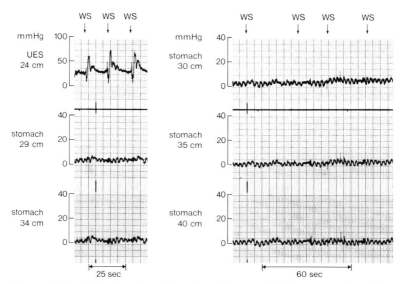

Figure 10-8.   Motor function of intrathoracic stomach following esophageal resection. UES function is normal. The interposed stomach has positive resting pressure despite its location in the chest. No gastric motor activity is observed with swallows. (WS, wet swallow.)

10–8). Voluntary swallows do not propagate through the anastomosed gastric remnant. Gastric activity, mainly type I waves, may be observed. An intact upper esophageal sphincter opposes the pressure present in the vagotomized gastric pouch and is an important prerequisite to prevent oral regurgitation and aspiration.[99]

With these considerations in mind, an "inkwell" type of anastomosis may be performed to prevent reflux. Patients with this type of reconstruction, who possess an adequate pressure gradient at the esophagogastric junction, do not have reflux. Those without a pressure gradient may have symptomatic reflux.[100]

Isoperistaltic gastric tubes used by Postlethwait and colleagues[101] show normal function of the proximal sphincter and the proximal esophageal segment. The gastric tube below the anastomosis is either completely inert or shows spontaneous uncoordinated activity. The resting pressure in the gastric tube is slightly positive (Fig. 10–9 A,B, and C).

The reversed gastric tube shows an autonomic pattern with rhythmic contractions of 20 seconds every 3 minutes.[102]

If a free gastric tube transplant is used to replace a portion of the cervical esophagus, it does not participate in the propagation of esophageal peristalsis.[103]

Reconstruction with the Jejunum and Ileum

The small bowel may be used as an interposed segment for reconstruction of the resected distal esophagus. Free transplants of small bowel have also been used for reconstruction of the cervical esophagus. An intact vascular supply to the interposed jejunal segment is important for its function. When a single vessel is used, a higher resting pressure exists in the segment and may cause bolus obstruction. If two vessels are used, no significant obstruction occurs.[104] The jejunum is an elastic but nonperistaltic segment.[105] The type of contractions present in the small bowel substitute are type I waves that are recorded at a constant rate of 11/min.[99]

In patients with an interposed jejunal substitute, segmental nonpropulsive contractions with occasional peristaltic waves are seen. Occasionally the jejunum may be completely inert. The interposed bowel retains its peristaltic function if placed in an isoperistaltic position.[106]

The ileum transplanted as a free graft lacks normal peristalsis.[103]

Reconstruction with the Colon

The right and left colon may be used as an interposed esophageal segment when positioned in either an iso or antiperistaltic manner.

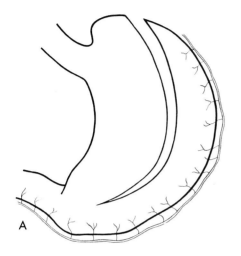

Figure 10-9. *A*, Isoperistaltic gastric tube fashioned from the greater curvature. *B*, Complete inactivity of the gastric tube in response to swallowing. (*WS*, wet swallow.) *C*, Spontaneous and disordered motor activity in the gastric tube in response to swallowing. (*DS*, dry swallow.)

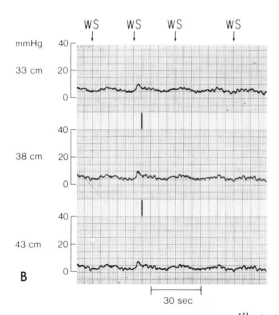

Illustration continues on opposite page

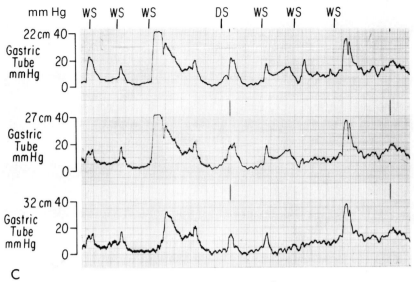

Figure 10-9C. *Continued.*

In some radiologic observations, no motor activity was observed in the interposed colon segments.[107] Motility studies also revealed that the colon has prolonged periods of inactivity[106] (Fig. 10–10). Others, however, reported that motor activity appears identical to that of the normal colon. Kelley concluded that even if the colon does not show a response to swallows, it can retain its ability to produce characteristic pressure deflections, albeit in an intrathoracic position.[97] Most observers do not mention true peristalsis in the interposed segment. In some studies, contractions of the transplanted segment are thought to keep the colon free of refluxed material. Maximal activity seems to be achieved in response to small acid loads. No high pressure can be detected at the distal anastomotic level.[108] The length of the colonic tube in the subdiaphragmatic position has been proposed as a major deterrent to reflux.[109]

The contractions of the colon are usually nonpropulsive. Sequential haustral contractions give the appearance of normal peristalsis. Transit is mainly passive and depends on gravity.[110] As in other types of esophageal reconstruction, the UES and normally functioning proximal esophagus are the major barriers to reflux. The hiatus and the distal anastomosis are useless in protecting against the positive pressure gradient from the abdomen. No transmission of peristalsis occurs between the esophagus and the transposed colonic segment.[111] Isoperistaltic interposition seems preferable because of monophasic local segmental contractions with peristaltic

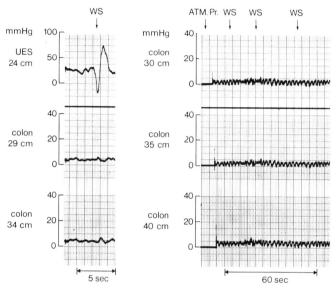

Figure 10-10. Full-length colon interposition. UES function is normal. The resting pressure in the colon is slightly positive. No colonic motor activity can be identified. (*WS*, wet swallow; *ATM. Pr.*, momentary opening of system to atmospheric pressure.)

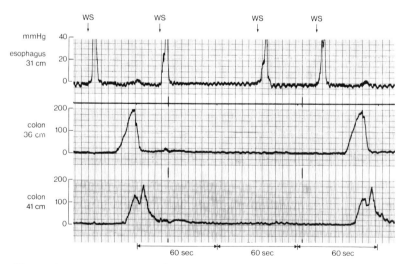

Figure 10-11. Motor activity of a short colon interposition used to replace the distal half of the esophagus. Esophageal peristalsis is not transmitted into the colonic segment. In this case, however, strong peristaltic contractions are observed in the colon. (*WS*, wet swallow.)

responses to acid perfusion. This may be a useful surgical modification to prevent reflux (Fig. 10–11).

Free colon transplants show nonpropulsive segmental activity.[103]

In summary, experimental as well as clinical observations suggest that the most appropriate substitute for the esophagus is an isoperistaltic one. Surgical measures should be carried out to preserve maximally the available vascular supply. The UES and proximal esophagus should be protected, and reflux of bile or acid in the interposed segment must be diminished.

REFERENCES

1. Welsh G. F., Payne W. S.: The present status of one-stage pharyngoesophageal diverticulectomy. Surg. Clin. North Am., 53:953–958, 1973.
2. Pedersen S. A., Hansen J. B., Alstrup P.: Pharyngo-oesophageal diverticula. A manometric follow-up study of ten cases treated by diverticulectomy. Scand. J. Thorac. Cardiovasc. Surg., 7:87–90, 1973.
3. Hurwitz A. L., Duranceau A.: Upper esophageal sphincter dysfunction pathogenesis and treatment. Am. J. Dig. Dis., 23:275–281, 1978.
4. Ellis H. F., Schlegel J. F., Lynch V. P., Payne W. S.: Cricopharyngeal myotomy for pharyngoesophageal diverticulum. Ann. Surg., 170:340–349, 1969.
5. Duranceau A., Letendre J., Clermont R., Lévesque H. P., Barbeau A.: Oropharyngeal dysphagia in patients with oculopharyngeal muscular dystrophy. Can. J. Surg., 21:326–329, 1978.
6. Henderson R. D., Woolf C., Marryatt G.: Pharyngoesophageal dysphagia and gastroesophageal reflux. Laryngoscope, 86:1531–1538, 1976.
7. Henderson R. D., Marryatt G.: Cricopharyngeal myotomy as a method of treating cricopharyngeal dysphagia secondary to gastroesophageal reflux. J. Thorac. Cardiovasc. Surg., 74:721–725, 1977.
8. Mansson I., Sandberg N.: Effects of surface anesthesia on deglutition in man. Laryngoscope, 84:427–437, 1974.
9. Henderson R. D., Boszko A., VanNostrand A. W. P.: Pharyngoesophageal dysphagia and recurrent laryngeal nerve palsy. J. Thorac. Cardiovasc. Surg., 68:507–112, 1974.
10. Duranceau A., Jamieson G., Hurwitz A. L., Jones R. S., Postlethwait R. W.: Alteration in esophageal motility after laryngectomy. Am. J. Surg., 131:30–35, 1976.
11. Dey F. L., Kirchner J. A.: The upper esophageal sphincter after laryngectomy. Laryngoscope, 71:99–115, 1961.
12. Mansson I., Sandberg N.: Manometry of the pharynx and the esophagus in relation to laryngectomy. J. Fr. Otorhinolaryngol., 23:737–743, 1974.
13. Lauerma K. S. L., Harvey J. E., Ogura J. H.: Cricopharyngeal myotomy in subtotal supraglottic laryngectomy: an experimental study. Laryngoscope, 82:447–453, 1972.
14. Winans C. S., Reichbach E. J., Waldrop W. F.: Esophageal determinants of alaryngeal speech. Arch. Otolaryngol., 99:10–14, 1974.
15. Bonanno P. C.: Swallowing dysfunction after tracheostomy. Ann Surg., 174:29–33, 1971.
16. Cohen S. , Harris L.: Does hiatus hernia affect competence of the gastroesophageal sphincter? N. Engl. J. Med., 284:1053–1056, 1971.
17. Behar J., Biancani P., Sheahan D. G.: Evaluation of esophageal tests in the diagnosis of reflux esophagitis. Gastroenterology, 71:9–15, 1976.
18. Olsen A. M., Schlegel J. F., Payne W. S.: The hypotensive gastroesophageal sphincter. Mayo Clin. Proc., 48:165–172, 1973.
19. Henderson R. D., Mugashe F., Jeejeebhoy K. N., Cullen J., Szczpanski M., Boszko A., Marryatt G.: The motor defect of esophagitis. Can. J. Surg., 17:112–116, 1974.

20. Henderson R. D., Mugashe F., Jeejeebhoy K. N., Cullen J., Szczepanski M., Boszko A., Marryatt G.: The role of bile and acid in the production of esophagitis and the motor defects of esophagitis. Ann. Thorac. Surg., 14:465–473, 1972.

21. Siegel C. I., Hendrix T. R.: Esophageal motor abnormalities induced by acid perfusion in patients with heartburn. J. Clin. Invest., 42:686–695, 1963.

22. Olsen A. M., Schlegel J. F.: Motility disturbances caused by esophagitis. J. Thorac. Cardiovasc. Surg., 50:607–612, 1965.

23. Henderson R. D., Pearson F. G.: Preoperative assessment of esophageal pathology. J. Thorac. Cardiovasc. Surg., 72:512–517, 1976.

24. Michelson E., Siegel C. I.: The role of the phrenico-esophageal ligament in the lower esophageal sphincter. Surg. Gynecol. Obstet. 118:1291–1294, 1964.

25. Khan T. A., Crispin J. S., Lind J. F.: Effect of change of position on the function of the canine lower esophageal sphincter. Gastroenterology, 67:957–964, 1974.

26. Khan T. A., Garzo V. G.: Evaluation of posterior gastropexy for gastroesophageal reflux. Arch. Surg., 112:623–626, 1977.

27. Allison P. R.: Hiatus hernia (a 20 year retrospective survey). Ann. Surg., 178:273–276, 1973.

28. Collis J. L.: Surgical control of reflux in hiatus hernia. Am. J. Surg., 115:465–471, 1968.

29. Habibulla K. S., Collis J. L.: Intraluminal pressure, transmucosal potential difference and pH studies in the esophagus of patients before and after Collis repair of a hiatal hernia. Thorax, 28:342–348, 1973.

30. Csendes A., Larrain A.: Effects of posterior gastropexy on gastroesopheageal sphincter pressure and symptomatic reflux in patients with hiatal hernia. Gastroenterology, 63:19–24, 1972.

31. Larrain A., Csendes A., Uribe P., Ayala M.: Manometric evaluation after posterior gastropexy for treatment of strictures of the esophagus secondary to reflux. Surg. Gynecol. Obstet., 136:564–566, 1973.

32. Lipshutz W. H., Eckert R. J., Gaskins R. D., Blanton D. E., Lukash W. M.: Normal lower esophageal sphincter function after surgical treatment of gastroesophageal reflux. N. Engl. J. Med., 291:1107–1110, 1974.

33. Dimarino A. J., Rosato E., Rosato F., Cohen S.: Improvement in lower esophageal sphincter pressure following surgery for complicated gastroesophageal reflux. Ann. Surg., 181:239–242, 1975.

34. Hill L. D.: Digestive Disease Week, Toronto, May 1977.

35. Skinner D. B., DeMeester T. R.: Gastroesophageal reflux. Curr. Probl. Surg., 13:1–62, 1976.

36. Alday E. S., Goldsmith H. S.: Efficacy of fundoplication in preventing gastric reflux. Am. J. Surg., 126:322–324, 1973.

37. Ellis F. H., El-Kurd M. F. A., Gibb S. P.: The effect of fundoplication on the lower esophageal sphincter. Surg. Gynecol. Obstet., 143:1–5, 1976.

38. Battle W. S., Nyhus L. M., Bombeck C. T.: Nissen fundoplication and esophagitis secondary to gastroesophageal reflux. Arch. Surg., 106:588–592, 1973.

39. DeMeester T. R., Johnson L. F., Kent A. H.: Evaluation of current operations for the prevention of gastroesophageal reflux. Ann. Surg., 180:511–525, 1974.

40. DeMeester T. R., Johnson L. F.: Evaluation of the Nissen antireflux procedure by esophageal manometry and twenty-four hour pH monitoring. Am. J. Surg., 129:94–100, 1975.

41. Bushkin F. L., Neustein C. L., Parker T. H., Woodward E. R.: Nissen fundoplication for reflux peptic esophagitis. Ann. Surg., 185:672, 1977.

42. Condon R. E., Kraus M. A., Wollheim D.: Cause of increase in "lower esophageal sphincter" pressure after fundoplication. J. Surg. Res., 20:445–450, 1976.

43. Bowes K. L., Sarna S. K.: Effect of fundoplication on the lower esophageal sphincter. Can. J. Surg., 18:328–333, 1975.

44. Siewert R., Jennewein H. M., Waldeck F., Peiper H. J.: Manometric investigations for reconstruction (fundoplication) of the lower esophageal sphincter in man and dog. In: The Function of the Esophagus. Odense University Press, Denmark, 1973.

45. Fisher R. S., Malmud L. S., Lobis I. F., Maier W. P.: Lower esophageal sphincter pressures and gastroesophageal reflux before and after fundoplication. Is there a correlation? Gastroenterology, 70:976, 1976.
46. Polk H. C.: Fundoplication for reflux esophagitis: misadventures with the operation of choice. Ann. Surg., 183:645–652, 1976.
47. Behar J., Sheahan D. G., Biancani P., Spiro H. M., Storer E. H.: Medical and surgical management of reflux esophagitis: a 38-month report on a prospective clinical trial. N. Engl. J. Med., 293:263–268, 1975.
48. Higgs R. H., Castell D. O., Farrell R. L.: Evaluation of the effect of fundoplication on the incompetent lower esophageal sphincter. Surg. Gynecol. Obstet., 141:571–575, 1975.
49. Behar, J., Biancani P., Spiro H. M., Storer E. H.: Effect of an anterior fundoplication on lower esophageal sphincter competence. Gastroenterology, 67:209–215, 1974.
50. Orringer M. B., Skinner D. B., Belsey R. H. R.: Long term results of the Mark IV operation for hiatal hernia and analyses of recurrences and their treatment. J. Thorac. Cardiovasc. Surg., 63:25–33, 1972.
51. Henderson R. D., Pearson F. G.: Surgical management of esophageal scleroderma. J. Thorac. Cardiovasc. Surg., 66:686–692, 1973.
52. Cooper J. D., Gill S. S., Nelems J. M., Pearson F. G.: Intraoperative and postoperative esophageal manometric findings with Collis gastroplasty and Belsey hiatal hernia repair for gastroesophageal reflux. J. Thorac. Cardiovasc. Surg. 74:744–751, 1977.
53. Henderson, R. D.: Reflux control following gastroplasty. Ann. Thorac. Surg., 24:206–214, 1977.
54. Thal A. P.: A unified approach to surgical problems of the esophagogastric junction. Ann. Surg., 168:542–550, 1968.
55. Jones F. L., Booth D. J., Cameron J. L., Zuidema G. D., Skinner D. B.: Functional evaluation of esophageal reconstructions. Ann. Thorac. Surg., 12:331–346, 1971.
56. Hollenbeck J. I., Woodward E. R.: Treatment of peptic esophageal stricture with combined fundic patch fundoplication. Ann. Surg., 182:472–477, 1975.
57. Balison J. R., MacGregor A. M. C., Woodward E. R.: Postoperative diaphragmatic herniation following transthoracic fundoplication. Arch. Surg., 106:164–166, 1973.
58. Woodward E. R.: Personal Communication. Am. Coll. Surg. Meeting, Dallas, Texas, 1977.
59. Ellis F. H., Kiser J. C., Schlegel J. F., Earlam R. J., McVey J. L., Olsen A. M.: Esophagomyotomy for esophageal achalasia; experimental, clinical and manometric aspects. Ann. Surg., 166:640–656, 1967.
60. McVey J. L., Schlegel J. F., Ellis F. H.: Gastroesophageal sphincteric function after the Heller myotomy and its modifications. An experimental study. Bull. Soc. Int. Chir. 22:419–423, 1963.
61. Mann C. V., Ellis F. H., Schlegel J. F., Code C. F.: Abdominal displacement of the canine G.E. sphincter. Surg. Gynecol. Obstet., 118:1009–1018, 1964.
62. Atkinson M.: The oesophagogastric sphincter after cardiomyotomy. Thorax, 14:125–131, 1959.
63. Vantrappen G., Van Goidsenhoven G. E., Verbeke S., Van Den Berghe G., Vandenbroucke J.: Manometric studies in achalasia of the cardia, before and after pneumatic dilations. Gastroenterology, 45:317–325, 1963.
64. Van Goidsenhoven G., Vantrappen G., Verbeke S., Vandenbroucke J.: Treatment of achalasia of the cardia with pneumatic dilations. Gastroenterology, 45:326–334, 1963.
65. Sanderson D. R., Ellis F. H., Olsen A. M.: Achalasia of the esophagus: results of therapy by dilatation, 1950–1967. Chest, 58:116–121, 1970.
66. Crump A. C., Flood C. A., Hennig G. C.: Results of medical treatment of idiopathic cardiospasm. Gastroenterology, 20:30–38, 1952.
67. Sultan M., Norton R. A.: Esophageal diameter and the treatment of achalasia. Am. J. Dig. Dis., 14:611–618, 1969.
68. Belsey R.: Disorders of function of the esophagus. In Surgery of the Esophagus. (R. A. Smith, R. E. Smith, eds.) The Coventry Conference, 1971. Butterworths, London.

69. Jekler J., Lhotka J.: Modified Heller procedure to prevent postoperative reflux esophagitis in patients with achalasia. Am. J. Surg., 113:251–254, 1967.

70. Ellis F., Cole F. L.: Reflux after cardiomyotomy. Gut, 6:80–84, 1965.

71. Black J., Vorbach A. N., Collis J. L.: Results of Heller's operation for achalasia of the esophagus: the importance of hiatal hernia repair. Br. J. Surg., 63:949–953, 1976.

72. DiMarino A. J., Cohen S.: Characteristics of lower esophageal sphincter function in symptomatic diffuse esophageal spasm. Gastroenterology, 66:1–6, 1974.

73. Paris F. , Benages A., Berenguer J., Blasco E., Garrido G., Parilla P., Ridocci M. T., Carbonell C.: Pre-and postoperative manometric studies in diffuse esophageal spasm. J. Thorac. Cardiovasc. Surg., 70:126–132, 1975.

74. Leonardi H. K., Shea J. A., Crozier R. E., Ellis F. H.: Diffuse spasm of the esophagus, clinical, manometric and surgical considerations. J. Thorac. Cardiovasc. Surg., 74:736–743, 1977.

75. Hurwitz A. L., Way L. W., Haddad J. K.: Epiphrenic diverticulum in association with an unusual motility disturbance: report of surgical correction. Gastroenterology, 68:795–798, 1975.

76. Henderson R. D., Pearson F. G.: Reflux control following extended myotomy in primary disordered motor activity (diffuse spasm) of the esophagus. Ann. Thorac. Surg., 22:278–283, 1976.

77. Higgs B., Kerr F. W., Ellis F. H.: The experimental production of esophageal achalasia by electrolytic lesions in the medulla. J. Thorac. Cardiovasc. Surg., 50:613–625, 1965.

78. Higgs B., Ellis F. H.: The effect of bilateral supranodosal vagotomy on canine esophageal function., Surgery, 58:828–834, 1965.

79. Burgess J. N., Schlegel J. F., Ellis F. H.: The effect of denervation on feline esophageal function and morphology. J. Surg. Res., 12:24–33, 1972.

80. Binder H. J., Bloom D. L., Stern H., Solitare G. B., Thayer W. R., Spiro H.M.: The effect of cervical vagectomy on esophageal function in the monkey. Surgery, 64:1075–1083, 1968.

81. Mann C. V., Code C. F., Schlegel J. F., Ellis F. H.: Intrinsic mechanisms controlling the mammalian gastroesophageal sphincter deprived of extrinsic nerve supply. Thorax, 23:634–639, 1968.

82. Burgess J. N., Kelly K. A., Schlegel J. F., Ellis F. H.: Effect of esophageal mucosal denervation on the motility of the canine esophagus. J. Surg. Res., 9:605–610, 1969.

83. Greenwood R. K., Schlegel J. F., Code C. F., Ellis F. H.: The effects of sympathectomy, vagotomy and esophageal interruption on the canine gastroesophageal sphincter. Thorax, 17:310–319, 1962.

84. Clarke S. B., Penry J. B., Ward P.: Esophageal reflux after abdominal vagotomy. Lancet, 2:824–826, 1965.

85. Crispin J. S., McIver D. K., Lind J. F.: Manometric study of the effect of vagotomy on the gastroesophageal sphincter. Can. J. Surg., 10:299–303, 1967.

86. Mazur J. M., Skinner D. B., Jones E. L., Zuidema G. D.: Effect of transabdominal vagotomy on the human gastroesophageal high pressure zone. Surgery, 73:818–822, 1973.

87. Johnston D.: Symposium on peptic ulcer. Laval University, Quebec City, November, 1975.

88. Khan T. A.: Effect of highly selective vagotomy on the lower esophageal sphincter. Ann. R. Coll. Surg. Can., 10:51, 1977.

89. Khan T. A., Crispin J. S.: Effect of highly selective vagotomy on the human lower esophageal sphincter (LES). Ann. R. Coll. Surg. Can., 11:49, 1978.

90. Mann C. V., Hardcastle J. D.: The effect of vagotomy on the human gastroesophageal sphincter. Gut, 9:688–695, 1968.

91. Thomas P. A., Earlam R. J.: The gastroesophageal junction before and after operations for duodenal ulcer. Br. J. Surg., 60:717–719, 1973.

92. Higgs R. H., Castell D. O.: Cholinergic stimulation of the lower esophageal sphincter in patients with vagotomy and antrectomy. Am. J. Dig. Dis. 20:195–200, 1975.

93. Haller J. A., Brooker A. F., Talber J. L., Baghdassarian O., Van Houtte J.: Esophageal function following resection. Ann. Thorac. Surg., 2:180–187, 1966.

94. Duranceau A., Fisher S. R., Flye M. W., Jones R. S., Postlethwait R. W., Sealy W. C.: Motor function of the esophagus after repair of esophageal atresia and tracheoesophageal fistula. Surgery, 82:116–123, 1977.

95. Lind J. F., Blanchard F. J., Guyda H.: Esophageal motility in tracheoesophageal fistula and esophageal atresia. Surg. Gynecol. Obstet., 123:557–564, 1966.

96. Janssens J., Valembois P., Pelemans W., Hellemans J., Vantrappen G.: Afferent impulses and primary esophageal peristalsis in the dog esophagus. In: *The Function of the Esophagus.* Odense University Press, Denmark, 1973.

97. Kelley M. L.: Intraluminal manometry in the evaluation of malignant disease of the esophagus. Cancer, 21:1011–1018, 1968.

98. Beschel H., Beck I.T.: Esophageal pressure studies in patients with carcinoma of the esophagus. Can. J. Surg., 17:211–216, 1974.

99. Miller H., Lam K. H., Ong G. B.: Observations of pressure waves in stomach, jejunal, and colonic loops used to replace the esophagus. Surgery, 78:543–551, 1975.

100. Pearson F. G., Henderson R. D., Parrish R. M.: An operative technique for the control of reflux following esophagogastrostomy. J. Thorac. Cardiovasc. Surg., 58:668–677, 1969.

101. Postlethwait R. W., Duranceau A.: Personal observations, 1978.

102. Gavriliu D.: Aspects of esophageal surgery. Curr. Probl. Surg., 12:1–64, 1975.

103. Hopkins D. M., Bernatz P. E.: Experimental replacement of the cervical esophagus. Arch. Surg., 87:265–275, 1963.

104. Jenkins D. H. R., MacLeod I. B.: Some observations on the behavior of isolated and interposed jejunal and ileal segments in the rabbit. Br. J. Surg., 57:835–840, 1970.

105. Williams G. S., Ingram P. R.: A comparative intraluminal oncometric study of the experimentally reconstructed esophagogastric junction. Surg. Gynecol. Obstet., 118:1205–1216, 1964.

106. Marshall R.: The results of laboratory and cine radiographic investigations after esophageal resection. In: *Surgery of the Esophagus.* (R. A. Smith, R. E. Smith, eds.) The Coventry Conference, Butterworths, London, 1971.

107. Belsey R. H.: Reconstruction of the esophagus with left colon. J. Thorac. Cardiovasc. Surg., 49:33–55, 1965.

108. Jones E. L., Booth D. J., Cameron J. L., Zuidema G. D., Skinner D. B.: Functional evaluation of esophageal reconstructions. Ann. Thorac. Surg., 12:331–346, 1971.

109. Henderson R. D., Fung K., Dube P., Marryatt G.: Esophageal reconstruction: an experimental approach to control of reflux after esophageal resection. Can. J. Surg., 18:165–169, 1975.

110. Clark J., Moraldi A., Moossa A. R., Hall A. W., DeMeester T. R., Skinner D. B.: Functional evaluation of the interposed colon as an esophageal substitute. Ann. Surg., 183:93–100, 1976.

111. Corazziari E., Mineo T. C., Anzini F., Torsoli A., Ricci C.: Functional evaluation of colon transplants used in esophageal reconstruction. Am. J. Dig. Dis., 22:7–12, 1977.

INDEX

Note: Page numbers in *italics* refer to illustrations.
Page numbers followed by (t) refer to tables.